DESIGNING AND CREATING A CULTURE OF CARE FOR STUDENTS AND FACULTY

THE CHAMBERLAIN UNIVERSITY COLLEGE OF NURSING MODEL

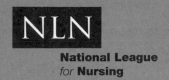

National League
for **Nursing**

DESIGNING AND CREATING A CULTURE OF CARE FOR STUDENTS AND FACULTY
THE CHAMBERLAIN UNIVERSITY COLLEGE OF NURSING MODEL

Edited by:

Susan L. Groenwald, PhD, RN, FAAN, ANEF

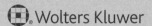

Philadelphia · Baltimore · New York · London
Buenos Aires · Hong Kong · Sydney · Tokyo

Executive Editor: Kelley Squazzo
Product Director: Jennifer K. Forestieri
Senior Development Editor: Meredith L. Brittain
Production Project Manager: Marian Bellus
Illustration Coordinator: Jennifer Clements
Manufacturing Coordinator: Karin Duffield
Marketing Manager: Katie Schlesinger
Prepress Vendor: Aptara, Inc.

Groenwald, S.L. (2018). *Designing and Creating a Culture of Care for Students and Faculty: The Chamberlain University College of Nursing Model.* Washington, DC: National League for Nursing.

9 8 7 6

Printed in The United States of America

Library of Congress Cataloging-in-Publication Data

Names: Groenwald, Susan L., editor. | National League for Nursing, sponsoring
  body.
Title: Designing and creating a culture of care for students and faculty :
  the Chamberlain University College of Nursing model / edited by Susan Groenwald.
Description: Philadelphia : Wolters Kluwer, [2018] | Includes bibliographical
  references.
Identifiers: LCCN 2017030870 | ISBN 9781496396211 (alk. paper)
Subjects: | MESH: Chamberlain University College of Nursing. | Models, Nursing |
  Education, Nursing | Schools, Nursing | Organizational Culture | United
  States
Classification: LCC RT73 | NLM WY 20.5 | DDC 610.73071/1—dc23
LC record available at https://lccn.loc.gov/2017030870

DRC0818

To our Chamberlain colleagues — who live Chamberlain Care *every day,
serving our students and each other.
And to our students — who chose us to partner with them on
their journey to becoming extraordinary nurses.*

About the Editor

Dr. Susan L. Groenwald is the president of Chamberlain University. She began her career as a rehabilitation nurse after earning a nursing diploma from West Suburban Hospital School of Nursing in Oak Park, Illinois. After earning bachelor's and master's degrees from Rush University College of Nursing in Chicago, Dr. Groenwald worked as a clinical nurse specialist and director of the oncology graduate program at Rush University and later served as the senior program director at the Illinois Cancer Council's Comprehensive Cancer Care Center. She earned a PhD in higher education leadership from Capella University. In 1981, Dr. Groenwald founded a company that provided 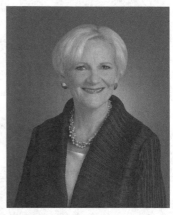 business-to-business services. Dr. Groenwald's accomplishments as a leader within the industry were recognized in 1999 when she was named National Businesswoman of the Year by the Chicago Chapter of the National Association of Women Business Owners and received a Blue Chip Enterprise Award from the U.S. Chamber of Commerce and Massachusetts Mutual. After selling the company, Dr. Groenwald served as the director of operations for Focused Health Solutions, Inc., developing clinical programs and managing a team of nurses who provided disease management services for large self-insured employers. In 2006, Dr. Groenwald joined Chamberlain University College of Nursing. She is the author of numerous articles and has edited five textbooks on cancer nursing, one of which—*Cancer Nursing: Principles and Practice*—won the *American Journal of Nursing* Book Award. Dr. Groenwald is a fellow of the American Academy of Nursing, the National League for Nursing's Academy of Nursing Education, and the Institute of Medicine Chicago.

About the Contributors

Kellie Bassell, EdD, MSN, RN, CNE is a faculty development specialist at Chamberlain University College of Nursing. She has more than 15 years of nursing education experience in both teaching and leadership across a variety of academic settings. She has participated in the development and implementation of imaginative and creative strategies to promote and support change in faculty's understanding of the teaching-learning process. She has authored and coauthored peer-reviewed journal articles and has presented at numerous higher education conferences across the United States. Dr. Bassell received a BSN from Boston College, an MSN from Florida Atlantic University, and a doctorate from the University of Florida.

W. Richard Cowling, III, PhD, RN, AHN-BC, FAAN, ANEF was most recently the vice president of academic affairs for Chamberlain University College of Nursing, where he helped shepherd the implementation of the *Chamberlain Care* Student Success Model. He is known for his academic leadership, including overseeing a 6-year major federal grant for promoting improved health care outcomes for diverse populations and creating a diverse faculty workforce. Dr. Cowling's most outstanding contributions have been in developing and applying a unitary appreciative nursing model to research and practice for women's survivorship of childhood abuse and depression. He has published and presented extensively through a variety of national and international venues. Dr. Cowling is the editor of the *Journal of Holistic Nursing*, and is certified as an advanced practice holistic nurse, and was named the 2008 Holistic Nurse of the Year by the American Holistic Nurses Association. He is a fellow in the American Academy of Nursing and in the National League for Nursing Academy of Nursing Education.

Carole R. Eldridge, DNP, RN, CNE, NEA-BC is the vice president of postlicensure and graduate programs for Chamberlain University, where she oversees Chamberlain programs delivered primarily online. She has served as a nursing college dean or director in four schools and led one of the first fully online executive nursing leadership programs. Before entering academia, Dr. Eldridge was the chief executive officer of a national home care and hospice corporation. She is the author of four books on elder care, five nursing textbook chapters, and several professional journal articles.

Laura Fillmore, DNP, MSN, RN, CNE is the director of prelicensure programs at Chamberlain University College of Nursing and leads academic teams of curriculum, clinical and simulation, global health, academic success, and faculty development. Dr. Fillmore developed and implemented strategic initiatives including interprofessional prelicensure courses, a comprehensive faculty development program with emphasis on academic quality, and student-centered learning environments with reflection and active learning environments. Dr. Fillmore presided over the National League for Nursing Center of Excellence application and designation journey. She has coauthored several articles in peer-reviewed journals and has developed symposiums and podium presentations at international and national nursing and higher education conferences.

Linda Hollinger-Smith, PhD, RN, FAAN, ANEF is the senior director for institutional effectiveness and research at Chamberlain University. She leads the university's program evaluation, quality improvement, and academic research efforts. Dr. Hollinger-Smith has served as the principal investigator on several public and privately funded studies supporting gerontologic nursing education. She served as a managing editor on the sole peer-reviewed journal for the seniors' housing industry and serves on editorial review boards for several peer-reviewed nursing journals. Dr. Hollinger-Smith is a fellow in the American Academy of Nursing and the National League for Nursing Academy of Nursing Education.

Chad O'Lynn, PhD, RN, CNE, ANEF is the director of evaluation and innovation at Chamberlain University. Through the years, Dr. O'Lynn has served the nursing profession as a clinician, researcher, educator, evaluator, and aromatherapist. He is the author and coeditor of two books on men in nursing and has published numerous articles and book chapters on male nursing students, rural nursing, and the Dedicated Education Unit. Dr. O'Lynn is a fellow in the National League for Nursing Academy of Nursing Education.

Candice Phillips, PhD, RN, APRN, CNM, CNE is a faculty development specialist at Chamberlain University College of Nursing. Dr. Phillips brings her expertise in experiential learning, innovative teaching strategies, new pedagogies, and the delivery of content using educational technology to support development of excellent nurse educators. At Chamberlain and throughout the academic community, she is well regarded for her capacity to develop educators into engaged explorers of the teaching and learning process. Her many presentations and publications address the role of faculty development in transforming nurse educators and leading organizational change. In addition to her work in academia, Dr. Phillips has many years of experience as a board-certified nurse midwife.

Carla D. Sanderson, PhD, RN is the provost of Chamberlain University. Dr. Sanderson's career spans the health care, higher education, regulation, public policy, and leadership development fields as an executive, board member, and volunteer. She has given multiple presentations and workshops on a variety of topics across the United States and internationally. She has authored seven book chapters, and a chapter on ethical decision making in nursing is in its seventh edition.

Foreword from the Chamberlain University Board of Trustees Chair

In *Designing and Creating a Culture of Care for Students and Faculty*, Susan Groenwald and colleagues make a clear and compelling case for caring in nursing programs. No one can argue with that premise—and yet if that were the sole focus of the text, the book's impact would be minimal. Many books and articles advocate for care and caring in nursing education. However, what truly distinguishes this text, and the work it describes throughout Chamberlain University College of Nursing, is its thorough coverage of how caring can be operationalized—and made tangible—in all aspects of a school's mission, vision, people, processes, and practices.

Chamberlain Care is the foundation. As described in Chapter 1, *Chamberlain Care* was originally an initiative focused on service excellence and over time has evolved into a philosophy, conceptual framework, and way of being for how nursing students at all levels are educated. *Chamberlain Care* is based on the belief that if students are to be successful, nursing education must incorporate the ideals of care for self, care for colleagues, and care for students. As Carla Sanderson, Chamberlain's recently appointed provost, notes: "Today, faculty and students are pursuing a reciprocal relationship of care as the purposes of higher education are fulfilled—to enhance intellectual exchange between faculty and students, inspiring students to learn to think and question, affecting in faculty the desire to stretch and grow to meet students where they are and take them where they need to be."

Embedding a philosophy throughout a school of nursing is daunting, as many deans and academic leaders have found. It is particularly difficult in a school as large (20 campuses in 14 states) and complex (pre- and postlicensure and graduate programs; on-site for some programs, online for others) as Chamberlain. This year, enrollment equals approximately 30,000 students.

Yet this text offers a blueprint for action for faculty in any school of nursing. *Chamberlain Care* in Action describes the work done to (1) enculturate the faculty in the philosophy and equip them with the necessary developmental opportunities and resources and (2) offer comprehensive support to the students as they face both academic and nonacademic challenges. Concrete strategies, practical insights, vignettes, and lessons learned from their journey (which Chamberlain leaders forthrightly acknowledge is far from over) illustrate key points.

But does it work?

Prior to joining the Chamberlain Board of Trustees, I became deeply immersed in learning about *Chamberlain Care* and Chamberlain's programs; in meeting faculty, staff, and students; and in examining Chamberlain's performance. I was impressed that student satisfaction and colleague engagement are key metrics that are measured. Meeting with students at least annually, I have appreciated their candid and thoughtful responses as to what is working and what could be improved. They are committed to having a voice and making a difference. As we visit campuses, there is a notable respect and camaraderie among the faculty and between students and faculty. I am touched when faculty or staff stop me in the halls of the central Chamberlain offices or at professional meetings and tell me how proud they are to be part of Chamberlain, often offering some anecdote as to how they have been personally supported in doing their best work.

Definitive research to answer the question and assess the impact of *Chamberlain Care* is under way, just as fundamental self-evaluation, revision, and improvement processes are ongoing. In the meantime, Susan Groenwald and the Chamberlain team offer a bold, comprehensive, pragmatic, and aspirational vision of what nursing education can be.

Joanne Disch, PhD, RN, FAAN
Professor ad Honorem, University of Minnesota School of Nursing
Chair, Board of Trustees, Chamberlain University

Foreword from the Cleveland Clinic Health System Executive Chief Nursing Officer

In 2015, I proudly achieved one of the greatest milestones of my professional career: I earned my DNP degree from Chamberlain College of Nursing (now the Chamberlain University College of Nursing). Obtaining my DNP was something I had wanted to do for years, but like many who lead busy personal and professional lives, the timing was never right. When I finally realized the time was now or never, I looked for a higher education institution that would deliver on everything I wanted and needed in my DNP pursuit. I was impressed by Chamberlain's rich history, committed values, high standards, and extensive offerings, and I knew I could achieve my goal if I attended a respected, high-quality institution like Chamberlain. Thus, after little debate, my choice was clear, and I began my DNP journey.

In all honesty, I expected that my DNP experience would be rather challenging. After all, I was earning the highest degree of my career while continuing to fulfill my role as an executive chief nursing officer (ECNO) for the world-renowned Cleveland Clinic health system and its 22,000 nursing caregivers. I expected to have even earlier mornings and later nights than usual. I expected that my time with my husband and two kids might be less than I would prefer some days. I expected that the work would be intense. And I expected that I would really need to push myself.

But I also expected that my experience would be highly beneficial and, truthfully, career changing. I expected my instructors to be experienced and informative. I expected to receive a well-rounded, comprehensive education. I expected to be able to apply what I was learning in the classroom to my daily work environment. And I expected to grow and emerge a better nurse.

However, what I did not expect was how much those at Chamberlain College also wanted me to succeed. What I did not expect was the extent to which my professors cared or the degree to which I received incredible faculty support. What I did not expect was how diverse my experience would end up being. What I did not expect was having the opportunity to really learn from my fellow students, who came from a variety of clinical settings and roles from across the United States. What I did not expect was how these extra benefits would positively impact my own scholarly work, my leadership role at Cleveland Clinic, and the future of my professional nursing career.

Throughout my experience, I saw firsthand how Chamberlain College aims to instill in its students the values required to be an extraordinary nurse. This culture of service and care was so evident and familiar to me because not that long ago, the Cleveland Clinic Nursing Institute made it a priority to design and create a similar culture within our own nursing organization. We wanted our nursing caregivers to really believe in our mission; to get excited about coming to work and be engaged and compassionate; to see the value in our Professional Practice Model and practice according to it; and to truly live, eat, and breathe our "patients first" mantra and deliver on the promise our nurses make to deliver patients world-class care. We worked diligently to give our caregivers the tools and resources they needed to be successful—to be extraordinary—by aiming to create a culture of service, education, research, innovation, collaboration, and quality care. We focused on values that define nursing excellence, such as quality, innovation, teamwork, service, integrity, and compassion—and we made it a priority to ensure that our nursing caregivers knew their leadership team cared about them, their well-being, and their success.

As a student at Chamberlain, I could easily recognize the way in which the organization promoted values of nursing excellence in my own learning, like self-determination, accountability, confidence, and courage. I can also see the success of Chamberlain's efforts through the many, many Cleveland Clinic nurses who are currently enrolled in Chamberlain's programs or are Chamberlain University College of Nursing graduates. Subsequently, the work that Chamberlain College has done to design and create its own culture of nursing excellence through superior service and care is phenomenal. It is research driven, evidence based, strategic, and measurable—and it directly improves the culture of health care organizations and patient care worldwide. The caliber of nurses who graduate from Chamberlain College is the caliber of nurses we seek at Cleveland Clinic health system.

Over the past few years, I have had the opportunity to get to know Susan Groenwald, PhD, RN, FAAN, ANEF, the president of Chamberlain University College of Nursing and primary author of this text. She is a remarkable leader and nurse. In this book, readers will garner insight into the development and implementation of Chamberlain's integrated, holistic educational model, *Chamberlain Care*, which incorporates the core ideals of care for self, care for colleagues, and care for students.

Readers will obtain a thorough understanding of the model and how it is incorporated into Chamberlain's learning environment, including key highlights such as how appreciation and support help students thrive and unlock their potential, how engagement and collaboration between faculty and students foster accountability and self-determination in nursing practice, and how a learning environment that promotes and instills confidence impacts a nurse's professional identity. Readers will also get an inside look at how to promote teaching excellence within this culture of care. This includes how to shift from a culture of traditional academics to one that is care based and service oriented, how to make improvements in teaching practice, and how to support and guide faculty development. I encourage readers to use the pages that follow to both personal and professional benefit. I can promise that you will not be disappointed.

Kelly Hancock, DNP, RN, NE-BC
Executive Chief Nursing Officer
Cleveland Clinic Health System

Preface

This book describes a 7-year journey at Chamberlain University College of Nursing designed to create an organizational culture and work climate called *Chamberlain Care*, in which students *and* colleagues thrive, and students are cared for in a way that improves their chances of success, providing an advantage in attracting and retaining high-quality and effective faculty and staff.

The journey began when Chamberlain embarked on a customer service initiative in 2010. I had been a student and champion of service excellence in prior roles I had held in business, but in my role as college president, a belief had grown in me that students in higher education deserve a unique form of service. Some would argue that students are not customers and that customer service has no place in education. I disagree. As I studied and thought more about it, I realized that the best service we can provide to our students in higher education is to help them reach their dream of an education and a better life for themselves and their families. At Chamberlain University College of Nursing, what better service can we provide to our students and to society than to help qualified students be admitted into nursing school, guide them to learn and graduate, and nurture them to become extraordinary nurses?

It was clear from our college's data that we were not yet achieving the level of service to which we aspired. Student retention was not as high as it could be, not all students passed NCLEX on the first attempt, not all students were satisfied with the value of the education received for the money paid, and not all graduates were extraordinary. We knew that there were service and outcome gaps we could address. We also knew that quality improvement required discipline and commitment, and that to bring others along, we had to create a compelling vision and answer the question *why*. And because it is hard work to be excellent, we also knew that we had to create a work environment where people want to be, and one where they are inspired and engaged.

I was disturbed by what I was seeing in higher education in the United States in general—a dearth of student support and encouragement, and more value placed on faculty research than on faculty teaching at some colleges and universities. The prevailing stories in nursing practice and education about student incivility, workplace hostility, toxic work environments, lateral violence, bullying, and job dissatisfaction reinforced to me the reality that at colleges and universities, we are, for the most part, not taking good care of students, and we are too often creating or tolerating climates that are hostile to students and colleagues. Students in colleges and universities often must learn how to navigate an environment built for survival of the fittest. Many students lack preparation for that kind of challenge, as evidenced by the graduation rates for first-time, full-time students across all U.S. colleges and universities (U.S. Department of Education, 2016).

Clearly, there was an opportunity in higher education, and specifically in nursing education, to create a bold new vision of student service and student support. Chamberlain's hypothesis was that by modeling and teaching critical values while students are in nursing school, we would arm our graduates with the characteristics that would empower them to be leaders in creating positive, healthy work environments.

To achieve our vision of creating an environment in which students and colleagues thrive and students become extraordinary nurses, we shaped and drove a culture of care that incorporates the concepts of care for self, care for colleagues, and care for students. What started as a quality improvement initiative drove a new vision, mission, and purpose for Chamberlain University College of Nursing, making us who we are today.

My colleagues and I have ourselves been transformed by our work together on this initiative and the results we have experienced. We designed this book to share our journey of how we catalyzed a culture of care and service throughout our organization and transformed our institution. Chapter 1 provides the reader a description and literature support of key concepts used in this book, including the concepts of culture, climate, care, and caring, and their impact on and importance to faculty and students. Chapter 2 begins with an overview of Chamberlain University College of Nursing to provide the reader context and then describes the six-phase transformational process that Chamberlain went through to create the *Chamberlain Care* Model. Chapter 2 includes vignettes and stories to give voice to those for whom *Chamberlain Care* has had an impact.

Chapter 3 addresses how *Chamberlain Care* both supports and honors faculty and staff at the same time it requires faculty excellence as a demonstration of care for students. In Chapter 3 is the history and results of our efforts to instill *Master Instruction* as our commitment to teaching excellence and student and faculty care. Chapter 3 also includes research findings evaluating the impact of *Master Instruction*, as well as assessing the degree to which faculty believe Chamberlain has a caring and supportive climate.

Chapter 4 focuses on the impact of *Chamberlain Care* on students and their success. Details of our first pilot under *Chamberlain Care* are provided, including evaluation data. The overall focus of Chapter 4 is the *Chamberlain Care* Student Success Model, which reflects our commitment to student success through the application of robust resources throughout the student life cycle, from admission to graduation and beyond. Also included in Chapter 4 is a discussion of how we are using data to drive decisions and initiatives, and to improve student success.

Finally, Chapter 5 reflects on the journey, lessons learned, and future opportunities and research.

Suggestions are included throughout the book, and Appendices A and B include tools that we hope might help others who embark on their own journey of cultural transformation. However, we understand that every institution is unique, with its own culture, mission, structure, people, and goals. Therefore, each journey of change will have its own set of challenges, pitfalls, and celebrations, and the methods and tools that we provide herein may have to be adapted.

We unabashedly advocate for more care in higher education, especially in nursing education, as a way to change the culture of the health care workplace. We also advocate that every leader—regardless of the size of the team, department, college, or system—pay attention to and deliberately create the desired culture that inspires and breeds loyalty. It does not have to cost anything but time, but the results can be remarkable.

We wish you an exciting, fulfilling, and challenging experience.

Susan Groenwald
President of Chamberlain University

"To infinity and beyond!"
—Buzz Lightyear in *Toy Story*

Reference

U.S. Department of Education. (2016). The condition of education 2016 (NCES 2016–144): Undergraduate retention and graduation rates. *National Center for Education Statistics*. Retrieved June 26, 2017, from https://nces.ed.gov/fastfacts/display.asp?id-40

Acknowledgments

We are grateful to Beverly Malone and Elaine Tagliareni at the NLN for the encouragement and opportunity to share our story.

Contents

1

The Case for a Culture of Care

Susan Groenwald, PhD, RN, FAAN, ANEF

Nurses and educators most often choose their professions because of their desire to help and care for people. Yet increasingly the literature is replete with articles and editorials about hostility in the workplace, nurses "eating their young," workplace violence, and incivility in educational and practice settings (Gallo, 2012; Hunt & Marini, 2012; Jones, Eschevarria, Sun, & Ryan, 2016; Lasater, Mood, Buchwach, & Dieckmann, 2015). Likewise, there is a preponderance of literature on incivility in nursing education particularly focusing on faculty behaviors (Clark & Kenaley, 2011; Clark, Olender, Kenski, & Cardoni, 2013; Newberry & Schaper, 2013). As health care agencies and educational institutions fight decreasing funding and resources, people tend to view their workplaces as mechanistic, devoid of fulfillment, or worse, hostile. Workers often believe that they are powerless to affect their work environment.

The same is true for students and their experiences in higher educational institutions, where there is often a lack of care and support. Many colleges greet students at freshman orientation with the phrase "look to your right, look to your left, in a year half of you will be gone." Colleges boast about "weeding out" students where only the strongest and most independent will survive, creating an environment of competition and fear.

Students are left to their own devices to figure out how to be successful. As a result, many students feel lost, lonely, confused, anxious, inadequate, and stressed. These problems lead to a high incidence of depression and anxiety among college students (Mahmoud, Staten, Hall, & Lennie, 2012). And yet research indicates that students do best when supported and encouraged (Jeffreys, 2014, 2015; Kareva, 2011; Noddings, 2016; Roberts & Styron, 2010). In fact, a Gallup (2014) survey of 30,000 college graduates showed that the odds of people thriving in their job and in their life more than doubled if the graduates had a professor in college who cared about them as a person, made them excited about learning, and encouraged them to pursue their dreams. The type of college or where they went to college hardly mattered at all—it was the caring provided by a faculty mentor that resulted in the difference. Sadly, less than a quarter of those graduates reported having such a faculty mentor in college. Clearly, there is room for more caring in higher education.

THE CASE FOR CARE IN HIGHER EDUCATION

Care and Caring

There are many definitions of care and caring—care as love, care as empathy, care as concern, interest, affection. A Google definition of the verb "caring" is "to display kindness and concern for others," whereas the noun *care* is "the provision of what is necessary for the health, welfare, maintenance, and protection of someone or something." Care theorists agree that the concepts of care and caring are multifaceted with varied interpretations and beliefs. For the Chamberlain initiative and model, the noun *care* was chosen to signify the outcome of the process of caring.

Noddings (2002) built on the care theory of Gilligan (1993), describing a relationship between caregivers and care receivers as entering into a mutually satisfying relationship in which both must agree to participate in the relationship. If the receiver fails to accept the caring, either because a relationship is lacking or the giver does not understand what the cared-for needs or cares about, then caring is not completed. Sumner (2001) described caring in nursing as "recognition of other and reciprocity" (p. 926). In her theory on human science and human care, Watson (2009) described care as both a value and an attitude, but asserted that the intention of caring is not enough—it is through concrete acts of caring that one cared-for can respond, but caring is complete only if and when the cared-for agrees.

Although *care* has different definitions in the classroom, all approaches to care involve teachers supporting students and providing them a sense of being cared for. Care in the classroom is a reciprocal relationship between students and faculty. Ladson-Billings (2009) demonstrated that students who were shown concern for their academic achievement and encouraged in emotional and social growth were engaged with their teachers, highly participatory in their education, and demonstrated high levels of academic scholarship and engagement. Noddings (2016) asserted, "Genuine education must engage the purposes and energies of those being educated" (p. 232).

Noddings (1988) applied the concept of caring to education and instruction and proposed four components in a model for moral education: modeling, dialogue, practice, and confirmation. Balmer, Hirsh, Monie, Weil, and Richards (2016) applied Noddings' philosophy to medical education, proposing that medical student interactions with teaching faculty would be caring encounters if three conditions are met: (a) teaching faculty understand the situations of students and respond to their needs, (b) students recognize their teachers as caring and respond accordingly, and (c) contextual continuities of duration and space are sufficient for a relationship to develop. The authors suggested that a caring relationship with their faculty in medical school can help students learn to be caring physicians.

To achieve the ideal of person-centered care in nursing practice, nurse educators must teach students caring behavior (Barnsteiner, Disch, & Walton, 2014). There is substantial research to show that when nursing faculty model caring behaviors in their interactions with students, it affects the way students later practice their professions (Balmer et al., 2016; Clouder, 2006; Sitzman, 2010; Touhy & Boykin, 2008).

Care and Impact on Student Success

Soto (2005) reported higher levels of nursing student engagement and academic success when students perceived of the school as a "caring institution," which also led to student persistence (p. 859). Soto suggested that caring strategies "may liberate students … from school-wide policies and teaching practices that maintain a cycle of educational poverty" (p. 861). McEnroe-Petitte (2011) built a case for the relationship of faculty caring to nursing student success, especially at-risk students. She advocates that faculty portray caring in a variety of ways to foster respect, instill self-confidence, and offer assistance.

Nursing students succeed first by staying in school, graduating, and passing NCLEX®, but ultimately through deep learning and developing the knowledge, skills, and values that employers want in nurses they hire. Chamberlain colleagues believe that caring for students enhances deep learning and engagement and that a culture of care and service provides professional role modeling of the kinds of behaviors expected of professional nurses. When faculty and academic leaders model for nursing students the appropriate behaviors of care, respect, and professionalism, they create a culture that decreases incivility and fosters collaboration, respect, and cooperation. Ultimately, these values and behaviors enhance patient care. Increasingly, these are the kinds of behaviors that health care agencies want in the nurses they employ: nurses with values of service, caring, integrity, and professionalism—extraordinary nurses.

Care and Faculty Excellence and Engagement

There exists a crisis resulting from a shortage of quality faculty and academic leadership necessary to teach the more than 68,000 interested and qualified prospective students who were turned away from baccalaureate and graduate nursing programs in the United States in 2015 alone (American Association of Colleges of Nursing, 2016; National League for Nursing, 2016). Research has shown that it is faculty and how they teach and care for students that is the most critical factor in student learning and satisfaction (Kareva, 2011; Roberts & Styron, 2010). Therefore, a scarcity of important faculty resources requires all nursing schools to focus on recruiting, developing, and retaining quality faculty.

In a survey of more than 1,350 nursing educators conducted by University of Arkansas nurse researchers, support from institutional leadership was identified as the most important factor for faculty who were satisfied with their jobs and planned to stay in them (Lee, Miller, Kippenbrock, Rosen, & Emory, 2017). Disch, Edwardson, and Advan (2004) reported that training programs focused on improving teaching abilities or helping faculty acquire new teaching skills and strategies were identified by faculty as important retention strategies. Faculty training and development is one important strategy in demonstrating to faculty that the institution cares about faculty personal fulfillment and continuous learning. Chamberlain's approach to faculty retention through its culture of care is discussed in Chapter 3.

THE CASE FOR CULTURE

Culture can be thought of as the personality of an organization, exemplified in the behavior of the people inside the organization, including formal and informal, conscious and nonconscious, written and verbal rules, processes, communications, beliefs, and customs. Every organization has a culture, whether the people who live it realize it or not. Many leaders ignore culture, letting it take its own shape and form. Other leaders shape and nurture their organizations to attain a specific culture. Most people can conjure an image of a company with a palpable culture that attracts repeat customers. Companies like Southwest Airlines, Apple, Nordstrom, and Disney come to mind. Undoubtedly, the leaders of those companies were deliberate in creating the cultures they wanted people to experience, talk about, and return to.

Organizational culture and climate emerged as key topics in business during the 1980s and 1990s, giving birth to major works in the study of managerial and organizational performance, including Peters and Waterman's *In Search of Excellence* (1982), Schein's *Organizational Culture and Leadership* (1985, 2010), and Kotter's *Leading Change* (1996, 2012). Early theorists described culture and climate as overlapping but different concepts. Hoy (1990) differentiated climate as being psychological (shared perceptions), whereas culture is anthropological (shared norms and values). Schein (1985, 1996), an early expert on organizational culture, stated that norms, values, rituals, and climate are all manifestations of culture. It is easier to measure behaviors than values, so climate is the concept most often researched, although the terms are very close. Because the intention at Chamberlain University College of Nursing (2017) was to change organizational *culture* for the purpose of creating a specific *climate,* both terms will be used in this book to describe different elements of the process.

Culture, Climate, and Organization Performance

A strong and positive culture translates into a set of organizational values, processes, and goals that guide employee behavior and organizational decision making and create vitality in the workplace. Denison, Haaland, and Goelzer (2004) determined that companies with cultures that exemplified involvement and participation, consistency, adaptability, and mission were most likely to perform better than peers. Since culture became an important organizational measure in the early 1980s, many authors have found a relationship between culture and better business performance in a variety of industries, including education (Bailey, Madden, Alfes, & Fletcher, 2017; Flamholtz & Randle, 2011; Gebauer, Edvardsson, & Bjurko, 2010; Gordon & Di'Tamaso, 1992; Kotter & Heskett, 1992; MacNeil, Prater, & Busch, 2009; Ruben, DeLisi, & Gigliotti, 2016; Thapa, Cohen, Guffey & Higgins-D'Alessandro., 2013; Xenikou & Simosi, 2006).

Culture, Climate, and Employee Engagement

Engagement of employees at work is a key strategic issue for all leaders as organizations compete to recruit and retain top talent. Employees engage in an organization when their individual values and goals align with their perception of the organization's values and goals. In today's world, people want from their employers more than a paycheck or even career progression. Millennials, who will reach 75 percent of the U.S. workforce in the next two decades, are especially hungry for an opportunity to demonstrate a higher purpose of their work (Sabrina, 2017), but workers from all generations have been shown to yearn for meaning at work (Bfau, 2015).

Deloitte University Press (2017) published the results of a survey of 10,000 human resource and business leaders in 140 countries. Eighty percent of executives rated culture and employee experience as very important, but only 22 percent reported that their organizations were excellent at building a differentiated experience for their employees. Deloitte identified five factors that contribute to a positive employee experience: meaningful work, supportive management, positive work environment, growth opportunities, and trust in leadership (p. 55).

A recent Gallup report disclosed that 63 percent of U.S. workers are not engaged in their work (Gallup, 2017). According to Gallup, engaged employees feel connected to their employer and are passionate about their work. They actively look for ways to improve their organization's performance, whereas workers who are unengaged do not strive to improve performance and often adversely affect the performance of those around them. A strong culture where the organization is clear about its mission, goals, and values is more likely to lead to engaged employees, and an organization with engaged employees is more likely to have better performance (Bailey et al., 2017; Flamholtz & Randle, 2011; Xenikou and Simosi, 2006).

The stakes are high in nursing and health care where employee engagement can impact morbidity and mortality of persons cared for. Bargagliotti (2011) suggested that nurses are more likely to engage in their workplace when there is a high level of trust and autonomy. Wong and colleagues (Bamford, Wong, & Laschinger, 2012; Wong, Laschinger, & Cummings, 2010) demonstrated that authentic leadership, exemplified by self-awareness, relational transparency, ethical behavior, and balanced processing, created a climate of honesty, integrity, and high ethical standards and significantly improved both staff nurse engagement and the nurses' perceptions of the quality of care on their unit. Leaders play a key role in creating a climate that engages employees.

Culture and climate are significant factors in the satisfaction, engagement and retention of faculty and staff in institutions of higher learning (Duphily, 2011; Lechuga, 2008; Florenthal & Tolstikov-Mast, 2012). Research shows that both students' satisfaction with their educational experience and student performance are better when there are motivated teachers and a positive organizational culture (Florenthal & Tolstikov-Mast, 2012; MacNeil et al., 2009; Umbach, 2007; Umbach & Wawrzynski, 2005).

Culture, Climate, and Higher Education

Tierney (1988) conducted a year-long study of culture in higher education Institutions in the United States, concluding that organizations are shaped by strong forces that emanate from within: "An organization's culture is reflected in what is done, how it is done, and who is involved in doing it" (p. 3). Tierney pointed out that people often live within a culture without being aware of the historical processes, communication, and methods that become the culture, and it is only when someone wanders outside the norms or there is some collision of culture that people become aware of it.

Most of the work on climate and culture of schools has been at the K-12 level. Thapa et al. (2013) reviewed research in this area and found a significant relationship between school climate and culture and student achievement. Several studies have shown that school climate is directly related to academic achievement at all levels of schooling, including high school and college (MacNeil et al., 2009). The impact on student success and achievement is not only on the immediate schooling but seems to persist for years (Gallup, 2014; Thapa et al., 2013).

Watson (2001) warned that not providing a "hospitable school climate" (p. 4) may have a negative impact on student learning and success. Barth (2001) suggested that the first purpose of a school is to create and provide a culture that is hospitable to human learning. But what exactly is hospitable to human learning? Wang, Haertel, and Walberg (1997) reviewed 50 years of research on what helps students learn and found that direct influences such as quality and style of instruction, faculty student interactions, and classroom activities had more influence on student learning than nondirect influences such as student demographics, school organization, and state and local policies, which were the least influential on student learning.

Educational research supports a link between leadership and effective school culture (Deal & Peterson, 2016; Tierney, 1988; Waters, Marzano, & McNulty, 2003; Witziers, Bosker, & Kruger, 2003). Lakomski (2001) concluded that there is a causal relationship between the role of a leader and the learning of an organization and suggested that it is more likely for a school to achieve real and sustained change by changing the culture of the school rather than by simply changing the ways in which the school operates and functions. The culture and climate of the school affects student achievement, and conversely the school leader directly influences culture and climate. The leader's role is to create an academic climate that most effectively encourages and increases student achievement.

CHOOSING A DIRECTION: DRIVING A CULTURE OF CARE

When you come to a fork in the road, take it.
—Yogi Berra

Cultures can and do change, but it is not an easy process. Kotter (2012) described cultural change as a complex process that takes place in stages. Schein (2010) suggested that cultural change is a process that requires people to "unlearn" behaviors before they can learn new ones. Theorists agree that cultural change is a transformational process that requires establishing and communicating a vision; creating a common language; getting buy-in and commitment from others; operationalizing the change in terms of infrastructure, processes, and policies; and fostering sustainability.

Leaders change the culture of an organization when they perceive a gap between the desired and prevailing culture and have a compelling reason to remediate the gap. In a white paper summarizing interviews with leaders at health care agencies that had undergone cultural transformation, Kimball (2005) categorized five primary catalysts for change, although many leaders reported experiencing more than one catalyst (p. 12):

1. Burning platform/significant threat
2. External restructuring (e.g., after a merger or acquisition)
3. New facilities or technology
4. Passion to be better/the best
5. Visionary leadership (often new leaders skilled at creating and managing change).

In 100 percent of the cases reported by Kimball (2005), the organization's top leadership initiated the change effort. A significant role of a leader is to create an environment in which transformation is possible by aligning and engaging people with the vision. Leading a massive change initiative of any kind requires personal commitment and willingness to take risk. Leading a cultural change initiative is all of that, but it can also be personally transformative for the leader as the leader engages with colleagues, embraces new perspectives, and inspires others to change.

THE *CHAMBERLAIN CARE*® MODEL

At Chamberlain, the motivation to change was a passion to be better and to graduate extraordinary nurses. Our journey toward cultural transformation began in 2010 when we embarked on an organization-wide initiative toward service excellence. As an advocate for service excellence as a path to improved satisfaction and organizational outcomes, I was interested in learning how through improving student satisfaction, we might improve student engagement and academic outcomes.

My views on our approach to service excellence shifted when in November of 2011 a consulting firm presented an unpublished report to our executive leadership team on research they had conducted on student retention in higher education. The consultant claimed that the average retention for first-year college students across the United States is 50 percent, and that this figure has not changed substantially in the past 50 years despite major efforts to improve it. The consulting firm's research had found isolated departments/campuses/locations at colleges and universities where there had been phenomenal results, but they found no institution that had overall better results than the others, despite the institutions' claims of robust student support and retention strategies. The presenter claimed that where there were positive results, there was a committed leader who expected students to be successful, and who had implemented repeatable processes sustained through continued focus on the issue. The presenter provided examples in industries other than higher education where successful outcomes had been achieved through the systematic implementation of repeatable, sustainable, standardized processes and practices that made a difference. Such practices have made a significant impact in patient safety through operating room checklists (Gawande, 2010; Haynes et al., 2009), processes for medication administration, and the like. The processes were repeatable and sustainable and made a significant impact on decreasing errors and improving patient safety.

I took away from that presentation on retention two key messages that shifted my views about how a service initiative should be delivered at Chamberlain. One was that there are many well-intended initiatives and projects implemented, but they eventually fail because the processes are not sustainable or scalable, and/or the organization lacks the discipline to maintain focus on the initiative over time. Many employees begin to view initiatives launched by organizations as "the flavor of the month" as they watch initiatives fizzle out over time. An example is the operating room checklist process mentioned previously. Some hospitals lack sufficient rigor to ensure that the processes are followed by every operating room team despite overwhelming evidence of the efficacy of the process.

The second takeaway about student retention was something I already knew, but my perspective shifted to a new view of the link between service and student retention. I wrote these observations:

> Students attend college to change their lives and the lives of their families.

> The cost of students leaving college without the degree they sought is substantial to the student and to the educational institution.

> The best service a higher education institution can provide is to help students achieve their goals and dreams.

> Service excellence means student success; enhancing student success is excellent service.

During the same time period, Chamberlain engaged a third-party agency to help us formalize our brand platform and value proposition. We conducted numerous focus groups and surveys with current and prospective students and reviewed secondary research on the nursing education market. From this work, we identified three distinctive characteristics of our college. Students perceived that Chamberlain employed a student-centric approach, structured programs and resources to help students be successful, and fostered an environment that advanced patient care by modeling compassion and care for students. These three pillars supported our brand positioning. We heard from students that what Chamberlain provided was more than the verb form of *care;* it was the noun form. Chamberlain colleagues were providing care in the context of doing whatever was in their power to support the success of students. We progressed from the idea that Chamberlain *cares* to the concept that we provide *Chamberlain Care* to all students and colleagues, thereby enhancing their ability to thrive.

In April 2012, the Chamberlain leadership articulated the following key assumptions:

> Many students of Chamberlain have challenges that prevent them from being successful.

> By providing a caring and supportive environment, students are empowered to succeed.

> A supportive and caring environment begins with engaged caring colleagues.

> Engaged caring colleagues create a supportive caring environment that fosters student success.

> To achieve our vision of graduating extraordinary nurses who will transform health care worldwide, we must model the behaviors of an extraordinary nurse.

On the basis of our research with students and the articulation of key assumptions, the Chamberlain service initiative was named *Chamberlain Care,* and the following definition of it was established:

> Chamberlain Care is the excellent service we provide to each other and to students to help them achieve their goals and reach their dreams.

We chose to use the noun *care* to reflect our commitment to and responsibility for providing the resources necessary for student success. Our tag line reflects that commitment to care and to producing extraordinary nurses: *Extraordinary Care. Extraordinary Nurses.*

To achieve our vision, we needed to create an environment in which students could thrive and chose the concept of care to exemplify the desired climate. We believe that if we take extraordinary care of our students, they are more likely to be successful—motivated instead of demotivated, encouraged instead of berated—and that if we model the kinds of values and behaviors we want in professional nurses, students are more likely to develop those values and behaviors: supportive, nurturing, caring, compassionate. We believe that the very best service we can provide our students is to help them be successful—retain, learn, graduate, pass NCLEX, gain employment, further their careers, and become lifelong learners and leaders in nursing. We believe this to be a holistic endeavor supporting students through academic and life challenges faced in the pursuit of their education. We further believe that to provide this service, we must all work together as colleagues in whatever way we touch students' lives, whether direct or indirect.

As we embarked on the journey to intentionally transform our culture to one of care, we realized that we had to first create a culture where our employees could thrive, as unless our employees feel supported and cared for, they will not have the capacity or motivation to care for students in the way we envision. A model for transforming our culture to support student and employee success emerged from our beliefs and visions of care—the *Chamberlain Care* Model. We began an initiative to drive a culture of care and service throughout the organization so that it would be part of our DNA. *Chamberlain Care* embodies the essence of what we are about as expressed in our vision, purpose, and mission.

Figure 1.1 illustrates how the concept of care is woven throughout the organization, beginning with an emphasis on *care for self.* It is only when we care for ourselves fully

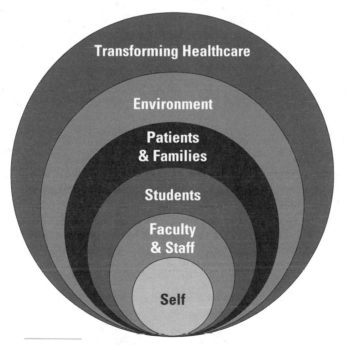

FIGURE 1.1 The *Chamberlain Care* Model: The power of 5 billion.

that we have the capacity to care for others. If we present our best selves at work, we are likely to be more caring, more productive, and more effective. This concept is touted in Ariana Huffington's book *Thrive,* in which she claims that in a relentless pursuit of success, American workers are exhausted, stressed, and unproductive (Huffington, 2014). When workers take care of themselves through proper rest, exercise, reflection, and regenerative activities, they are significantly more productive at work and in relationships. MacRae and Strout (2015) reported on a self-care project for faculty of future health care professionals to address the gap between self-care for health care providers and care and wellness of clients. The results of this small study demonstrated that when faculty and staff modeled self-care behaviors, their students took on and expanded self-care behaviors. Learning to practice self-care will inure to the benefit of nursing students' work and the clients they serve now and in the future.

The next part of the model is *care for colleagues,* which speaks to creating a respectful, supportive, and collegial environment where there is a shared vision and values. We made the decision as an organization to move away from the term *employee* and embrace the term *colleague.* It was not merely a change in language but a new appreciation of the nature of our work and an emphasis on collaboration and community. When people are inspired by what they do, and share the inspiration with others, amazing things can be accomplished. Creating community can be challenging in an educational environment where there is competition among faculty for promotion, tenure, or favorite assignments. In Chapter 3, we share our experiences and suggest opportunities for building communities of care among faculty and staff.

The next layer of the model is *care for students,* where we provide extraordinary care of students by providing resources and support to help students succeed. This concept is addressed in Chapter 4. The vision is that the extraordinary care modeled and provided at Chamberlain extends to the outer two circles in the model. Chamberlain graduates will provide care and service to the people for whose care they are entrusted and bring to their workplace values that can help transform health care worldwide. This extends across all forms of nursing practice and roles in nursing beyond practice such as education and leadership. Since Chamberlain offers programs across the prelicensure and postlicensure spectrum, we designed *Chamberlain Care* to support students in all programs of study.

Chamberlain has more than 40,000 nurse alumni and approximately 30,000 currently enrolled students. A network of 70,000 Chamberlain nurses in the world affecting health care is a powerful force. By using a hypothetical formula of a 30-year average work life of a nurse and approximately 10 average daily interactions with patients and families, we estimated that the 70,000 Chamberlain nurses will have more than 5 billion patient and family interactions over their careers. It is undeniable that those 70,000 Chamberlain nurses will have an impact. So why not be intentional and deliberate in creating an educational environment in which those Chamberlain nurses receive the very best education and are shown the path to the behaviors and values that extraordinary nurses exemplify?

The *Chamberlain Care* initiative evolved into a philosophy and conceptual framework and an integrated, holistic educational model that incorporates the core ideals of care for self, care for colleagues, and care for students. The College Guiding Statements, shown in Box 1.1, reflect our culture, values, and philosophy.

BOX 1.1

Chamberlain University Guiding Statements

Purpose: To create an academic culture in which colleagues and students thrive and that cultivates extraordinary graduates.

Mission: To educate, empower, and embolden diverse healthcare professionals who advance the health of people, families, communities, and nations.

Vision: By living *Chamberlain Care,* we graduate extraordinary nursing professionals who transform healthcare worldwide.

References

American Association of Colleges of Nursing. (2016). *2015–2016 Enrollment and graduations in baccalaureate and graduate programs in nursing*. Retrieved June 17, 2017, from http://www.aacn.nche.edu/leading-initiatives/research-data/E-G15toc.pdf

Bailey, C., Madden, A., Alfes, K., & Fletcher, L. (2017). The meaning, antecedents and outcomes of employee engagement: A narrative synthesis. *International Journal of Management Reviews, 19*, 31–53. Available at http://onlinelibrary.wiley.com/doi/10.1111/ijmr.12077/epdf. doi:10.1111/ijmr.12077

Balmer, D. F., Hirsh, D. A., Monie, D., Weil, H., & Richards, B. F. (2016). Caring to care: Applying Noddings' philosophy to medical education. *Academic Medicine, 91*(12), 1618–1621. doi:10.1097/ACM.0000000000001207

Bamford, M., Wong, C. A., & Laschinger, H. (2012). The influence of authentic leadership and areas of worklife on work engagement of registered nurses. *Journal of Nursing Management 21*(3), 529–540. doi:10.1111/j.1365-2834.2012.01399.x

Bargagliotti, L. A. (2011). Work engagement in nursing: A concept analysis. *Journal of Advanced Nursing, 68*(6), 1414–1428. doi:10.1111/j.1365-2648.2011.05859.x

Barnsteiner, J. H., Disch, J., & Walton, M. K. (2014). *Person and family-centered care.* Indianapolis: Sigma Theta Tau International.

Barth, R. S. (2001). *Learning by heart.* San Francisco: Jossey-Bass.

Bfau, B. N. (2015). How an accounting firm convinced its employees they could change the world. *Harvard Business Review.* Retrieved June 17, 2017, from https://hbr.org/2015/10/how-an-accounting-firm-convinced-its-employees-they-could-change-the-world

Chamberlain University College of Nursing. (2017). *Academic catalog.* Retrieved June 17, 2017, from http://www.chamberlain.edu/about/mission

Clark, C. M., & Kenaley, B. L. D. (2011). Faculty empowerment of students to foster civility in nursing education: A merging of two conceptual models. *Nursing Outlook, 59*(3), 158–165. doi:10.1016/j.outlook.2010.12.005

Clark, C. M., Olender, L., Kenski, D., & Cardoni, C. (2013). Exploring and addressing faculty-to-faculty incivility: A national perspective and literature review. *Journal of Nursing Education, 52*(4), 211–218. Available at http://www.healio.com/nursing/journals/jne/2013-4-52-4/%7Be3c88c65-36a2-4ef2-a8bb-723ca461fea9%7D/exploring-and-addressing-faculty-to-faculty-incivility-a-national-perspective-and-literature-review

Clouder, L. (2006). Caring as a 'threshold concept': Transforming students in higher education into health(care) professionals. *Teaching in Higher Education, 10*(4), 505–517. doi:10.1080/13562510500239141

Deal, T. E., & Peterson, K. D. (2016). *Shaping school culture.* New York: Wiley.

Deloitte University Press. (2017). Rewriting the rules for the digital age. *2017 Deloitte Global Human Capital Trends.* Retrieved June 17, 2017, from https://www2.deloitte.com/content/dam/Deloitte/global/Documents/HumanCapital/hc-2017-global-human-capital-trends-gx.pdf

Denison, D. R., Haaland, S., & Goelzer, P. (2004). Corporate culture and organizational effectiveness: Is Asia different from the rest of the world? *Organizational Dynamics, 33*(1), 98–109. doi:10.106/j.orgdyn.2003.11.008

Disch, J., Edwardson, S., & Adwan, J. (2004). Nursing faculty satisfaction with individual, institutional, and leadership factors. *Journal of Professional Nursing, 20*(5), 323–332. doi:10.1016/j.profnurs.2004.07.011

Duphily, N. H. (2011). The impact of culture on faculty retention in nursing education. *i-manager's Journal on Nursing, 1*(2), 1–8.

Flamholtz, E., & Randle, Y. (2011). *Corporate culture: The ultimate strategic asset.* Stanford, CA: Stanford Business Books.

Florenthal, B., & Tolstikov-Mast, Y. (2012). Organizational culture: Comparing faculty and staff perceptions. *Journal of Higher Education Theory and Practice, 12*(6), 81–90.

Gallo, V. J. (2012). Incivility in nursing education: A review of the literature. *Teaching and Learning in Nursing, 7*(2), 62–66. doi:10.1016/j.teln.2011.11.006

Gallup. (2014). Great jobs. Great lives. *The 2014 Gallup-Purdue Index Report.* Retrieved June 17, 2017, from https://www.lumina-foundation.org/files/resources/galluppurdueindex-report-2014.pdf

Gallup. (2017). *State of the American workplace.* Retrieved June 17, 2017, from http://www.gallup.com/services/178514/state-american-workplace.aspx?g_source=EMPLOYEE_ENGAGEMENT&g_medium=topic&g_campaign=tiles

Gawande, A. (2010). *The checklist manifesto.* Haryana, India: Penguin.

Gebauer, H., Edvardsson, B., & Bjurko, M. (2010). The impact of service orientation in corporate culture on business performance in manufacturing companies. *Journal of Service Management, 21*(2), 237–259. Available at http://dx.doi.org/10.1108/09564231011039303

Gilligan, C. (1993). *In a different voice: Psychological theory and women's development.* Cambridge, MA: Harvard University Press.

Gordon, G. G., & Di'Tomaso, N. (1992). Predicting corporate performance from organizational culture. *Journal of Management Studies, 29*(6), 783–798. doi:10.111/j.1467-6486.1992.tb00689.x

Haynes, A. B., Weiser, T. G., Berry, W. R., Lipsitz, S. R., Breizat, A-H. S., Dellinger, E. P., Herbosa, T., et al. (2009). A surgical safety checklist to reduce morbidity and mortality in a global population. *New England Journal of Medicine, 360*, 491–499. doi:10.1056/NEJMsa0810119

Hoy, W. K. (1990). Organizational climate and culture: A conceptual analysis of the school workplace. *Journal of Educational and Psychological Consultation, 1*(2), 149–168. doi:10.1207/s1532768xjepc0102_4

Huffington, A. (2014). *Thrive: The third metric to redefining success and creating a life of well-being, wisdom, and wonder.* New York: Harmony.

Hunt, C., & Marini, Z. A. (2012). Incivility in the practice environment: A perspective from clinical nursing teachers. *Nursing Education in Practice 12*, 366–379. doi:10.1016/j.nepr.2012.05.001

Jeffreys, M. R. (2014). Student retention and success: Optimizing outcomes through holistic competence and proactive student enrichment. *Teaching and Learning in Nursing, 9*, 164–170. doi:10.1016/j.teln.2014.05.003

Jeffreys, M. R. (2015). Jeffreys' Nursing Universal Retention and Success model: Overview and action ideas for optimizing outcomes A-Z. *Nursing Education Today, 35*, 425–431. doi:10.1016/j.nedt.2014.11.004

Jones, L., Eschevarria, I., Sun, E., & Ryan, J. G. (2016). Incivility across the nursing continuum. *Holistic Nursing Practice, 30*(5), 263–268. doi:10.1097/HNP.0000000000000167

Kareva, V. (2011). The influence of classroom communication on student commitment to the university. *European Scientific Journal, 7*(26), 90–104. Available at http://eujournal. org/index.php/esj/article/view/4626

Kimball, B. (2005). *Cultural transformation in healthcare: A white paper that describes the complex nature of organizational culture and its role in health care organizations.* Retrieved June 17, 2017, from https://folio. iupui.edu/bitstream/handle/10244/516/ NursingCulturalTrans.pdf?sequence=2

Kotter, J. P. (1996, 2012). *Leading change.* Boston: Harvard Business Review Press.

Kotter, J. P., & Heskett, J. L. (1992). *Corporate culture and performance.* New York: Free Press.

Ladson-Billings, G. (2009). *Dreamkeepers: Successful teachers of African-American children* (2nd ed.). San Francisco: Jossey-Bass.

Lakomski, G. (2001). Organizational change, leadership and learning: Culture as cognitive process. *International Journal of Educational Management, 15*(2), 68–77. doi:10.1108/09513540110383791

Lasater, K., Mood, L., Buchwach, D., & Dieckmann, N. F. (2015). Reducing incivility in the workplace: Results of a three-part educational intervention. *Journal of Continuing Education in Nursing, 46*(1), 15–24. doi:10.3928/00220124-20141224-01

Lechuga, V. (2008). Assessment, knowledge and customer service: Contextualizing faculty work at for-profit colleges and universities. *Review of Higher Education, 31*(3), 287–307. doi:10.1353/rhe.2008.0004

Lee, P., Miller, M. T., Kippenbrock, T. A, Rosen, C., & Emory, J. (2017). College nursing faculty job satisfaction and retention: A national perspective. *Journal of Professional Nursing.* doi:10.1016/j.profnurs.2017.01.001

MacNeil, A. J., Prater, D. L., & Busch, S. (2009). The effects of school culture and climate on student achievement. *International Journal of Leadership in Education, 12*(1), 73–84. doi:10.1080/13603120701576241

MacRae, N., & Strout, K. (2015). Self-care project for faculty and staff of future health care professionals: Case report. *Work, 52*(3), 525–531. doi:10.3233/WOR-152191

Mahmoud, J. S. R., Staten, R., Hall, L. A., & Lennie, T. A. (2012). The relationship among young adult college students' depression, anxiety, stress, demographics, life satisfaction, and coping styles. *Issues in Mental Health Nursing, 33*(3), 149–156. doi:10.3109/0 1612840.2011.632708

McEnroe-Petitte, D. M. (2011). Impact of faculty caring on student retention and success. *Teaching and Learning in Nursing, 6*, 80–83. doi.10.1016/j.teln.2010.12.005

National League for Nursing. (2016). NLN Faculty Census Survey 2014–2015. Retrieved June 17, 2017, from http://www.nln.org/ newsroom/nursing-education-statistics/ annual-survey-of-schools-of-nursing-academic-year-2015-2016

Newberry, S. M., & Schaper, A. M. (2013). Incivility in nursing education. *Journal of Continuing Education in Nursing, 40*(9), 403–410. doi:10755/291020

Noddings, N. (1988). An ethic of caring and its implications for instructional arrangements. *American Journal of Education, 96*(2), 215–230. doi:10.1086/443894

Noddings, N. (2002). *Educating moral people: A caring alternative to character education.* Williston, VT: Teachers College Press.

Noddings, N. (2016). *Philosophy of education* (4th ed.). Boulder, CO: Westview Press.

Peters, T. J., & Waterman, R. H. (1982). *In search of excellence.* New York: Harper & Row.

Roberts, J., & Styron, R., Jr. (2010). Student satisfaction and persistence: Factors vital to student retention. *Research in Higher Education Journal, 6*, 1–18. Available at http:// www.aabri.com/manuscripts/09321.pdf

Ruben, B. D., DeLisi, R., & Gigliotti, R. A. (2016). *A guide for leaders in higher education: Core concepts, competencies, and tools.* Sterling, VA: Stylus.

Sabrina, D. (2017). Rising trend: Social responsibility is high on Millennials' list. *Huffington Post: The Blog.* Retrieved June 17, 2017, from http://www.huffingtonpost. com/danielle.sabrina/rising-trend-social-respo_b_14578380.html

Schein, E. H. (1985, 2010). *Organizational culture and leadership* (3rd ed.). San Francisco: Jossey-Bass.

Schein, E. H. (1996). Culture: The missing concept in organization studies. *Administrative Science Quarterly, 41*(2), 229–240. doi:10.2307/2393715

Sitzman, K. (2010). Student-preferred caring behaviors for online nursing education. *Nursing Education Perspectives, 31*(3), 171–178.

Soto, N. E. (2005). Caring and relationships: Developing a pedagogy of caring. *Villanova Law Review, 50*(4), 859–874. Available at http://digitalcommons.law.villanova.edu/vlr/vol50/iss4/11

Sumner, J. (2001). Caring in nursing: A different interpretation. *Journal of Advanced Nursing, 36*(6), 926–932. doi:10.1046/j.1365-2648.2001.01930.x

Thapa, A., Cohen, J., Guffey, S., & Higgins-D'Alessandro, A. (2013). A review of school climate research. *Review of Educational Research, 83*(3), 357–385. doi:10.3102/0034654313483907

Tierney, W. G. (1988). Organizational culture in higher education: Defining the essentials. *Journal of Higher Education, 59*(1), 2–21. Available at http://faculty.mu.edu.sa/public/uploads/1360751907.3479organizational%20cult10.pdf

Touhy, T., & Boykin, A. (2008). Caring as the central domain in nursing education. *International Journal for Human Caring, 12*(2), 8–15.

Umbach, P. D. (2007). Faculty cultures and college teaching. In R. P. Perry & J. C. Smart (Eds.), *The scholarship of teaching and learning in higher education: An evidence-based perspective* (pp. 263–317). Dordrecht, Netherlands: Springer.

Umbach, P. D., & Wawrzynski, M. R. (2005). Faculty do matter: The role of college faculty in student learning and engagement. *Research in Higher Education, 46*(2), 153–184. doi:10.1007/s11162-004-1598-1

Wang, M. C., Haertel, G. D., & Walberg, H. J. (1997). *What helps students learn? Spotlight on student success*. Retrieved June 17, 2017, from http://files.eric.ed.gov/fulltext/ED461694.pdf

Waters, T., Marzano, R. J., & McNulty, B. (2003). *Balanced leadership: What 30 years of research tells us about the effect of leadership on student achievement*. Retrieved June 17, 2017, from http://files.eric.ed.gov/fulltext/ED481972.pdf

Watson, J. (2009). Caring science and human caring theory: Transforming personal and professional practices of nursing and health care. *Journal of Health and Human Services Administration, 31*(4), 466–482. Available at http://www.jstor.org/stable/25790743

Watson, N. (2001). "Promising practices": What does it really take to make a difference? *Education Canada, 40*(4), 4–6. Available at http://www.cea-ace.ca/sites/cea-ace.ca/files/EdCan-2001-v40-n4-Watson.pdf

Witziers, B., Bosker, R., & Kruger, M. (2003). Educational leadership and student achievement: The elusive search for an association. *Educational Administration Quarterly, 39*(3), 398–423.

Wong, C. A., Laschinger, H. K., & Cummings, G. G. (2010). Authentic leadership and nurses' voice behavior and perceptions of care quality. *Journal of Nursing Management, 18*(8), 889–900. doi:10.1111/j.1365-2834.2010.01113.x

Xenikou, A., & Simosi, M. (2006). Organizational culture and transformational leadership as predictors of business unit performance. *Journal of Managerial Psychology, 21*(6), 566–579. doi:10.1108/02683940610684409

2

Designing a New Model of Academic Service: Operationalizing *Chamberlain Care*

Susan Groenwald, PhD, RN, FAAN, ANEF

THE PROCESS OF CULTURAL TRANSFORMATION

Chamberlain pursued its objectives through a two-pronged approach to (1) Intentionally transform the institution's culture to one of care and service and (2) build the processes to support the desired culture of care to enhance student success. This chapter reviews the process in which Chamberlain engaged to develop a model, initiate a pilot to test the model, provide structure and accountability for continuous improvement initiatives that achieved our goals, and embark on a path to develop a culture of caring and service at Chamberlain.

Cultures change continuously as people within the organization change, but transforming an existing culture is not for the faint of heart. Driving cultural transformation requires changing peoples' beliefs, underlying assumptions, behaviors, and processes in a way that is deep and pervasive throughout the entire institution.

WHO AND WHAT IS CHAMBERLAIN UNIVERSITY COLLEGE OF NURSING?

So that readers can appreciate the complexity of the cultural transformation process at Chamberlain, the following section provides background on the university, the geographic distribution of students and faculty, and the size and scope of the university's operations. Chamberlain also has unique structures and processes that must be considered by others who may want to adapt an approach or tool to fit their organizations.

Deaconess School of Nursing was founded in 1889 in St. Louis, Missouri, and was acquired by Adtalem Global Education in 2005, at which time the name was changed to Chamberlain College of Nursing. Chamberlain is a regionally accredited institution of higher education that originally focused exclusively on nursing education. However, in May 2017, Chamberlain transitioned to a university structure with two colleges: the College of Nursing and the College of Health Professions. This book describes the process that took place within the College of Nursing before the transition to Chamberlain University.

Chamberlain University College of Nursing's enrollment as of April 2017 was just under 30,000 nursing students distributed among three degree levels and multiple program offerings. The prelicensure BSN program is delivered in a face-to-face format at 20 campuses in 14 states. Mature campuses range in size from 200 students to more than 1,000 students. The BSN is a year-round program that students complete in 3 years or less of full-time study. The curriculum is standard among campuses as required by our regional and professional accreditors. Courses are available in a standardized format in the learning management system so that students on every campus have the same syllabi, standard assignments, simulation experiences, and course resources. Of course, each campus has its own culture and personality, and it is the individual faculty who make the courses come alive for students in the classroom, where didactic information is applied in an active learning environment.

The focus of the faculty is teaching; 75 percent of their workload consists of teaching credits, and 25 percent of the faculty workload is split between scholarship and service credits. Chamberlain does not have tenure; all colleagues, including faculty, are employed "at will." Chamberlain has a rank and promotion system that enables faculty to advance by meeting criteria explicated for each rank. All full-time faculty have individual performance goals established with their manager at the start of the academic year and used for annual performance evaluation. Faculty and other colleagues also work with their leaders to create individual development plans for professional advancement. The average annual turnover of all full-time faculty declined for the third year in a row and was only 13.91 percent in fiscal year 2016 (Adtalem Global Education Human Resources Data System, 2017), which is under the 15 percent rate considered healthy for an organization (Kenny, 2007).

The prelicensure nursing student population at Chamberlain is highly diverse. Chamberlain participated in the 2016 annual survey of the American Association of Colleges of Nursing (AACN) and reported that 53.8 percent of the total population of students enrolled in the prelicensure BSN program as of fall 2015 came from a minority background compared to only 31.6 percent at other BSN entry programs at U.S. colleges of nursing (AACN, 2016). Over the same period, 13.6 percent of prelicensure BSN students at Chamberlain were male compared to 13.1 percent at other U.S. BSN programs. Although our faculty are not as diverse as our student population, 37 percent of the 322 full-time faculty are people of color compared to only 14.9 percent among other U.S. colleges of nursing; 8 percent of Chamberlain full-time faculty are male.

Chamberlain offers several postlicensure degree programs in a hybrid format, with most coursework online and clinical face-to-face using a typical practicum and/or immersion format. Postlicensure programs include RN-BSN, RN-MSN, and MSN with five specialty tracks (nurse educator, nurse executive, informatics, health care policy, and family nurse practitioner). Chamberlain also offers a hybrid DNP program focused on health care systems leadership.

As of April 2017, Chamberlain employed more than 1,220 full-time staff, including approximately 322 full-time faculty and 1,752 visiting professors (clinical and adjunct faculty). Classroom instruction on campuses is almost exclusively provided by full-time faculty; clinical instruction is a mix of full-time and adjunct faculty, but the majority of clinical faculty is part time. With faculty, students, and campuses distributed throughout the United States, change management is a complex process.

THE PHASES OF CULTURAL TRANSFORMATION

Chamberlain's journey to change attitudes, behaviors, and processes throughout the whole organization in a very intentional manner for transforming our culture is described in the following sections as having occurred in six phases. Although the six phases are presented sequentially, our actual experience was nonsequential; nonlinear; often messy; and full of surprises, challenges, and missteps. It is easy with hindsight to have clarity about what worked and what did not work, but the process was organic and unfolded as we went forward. In retrospect, we learned that all phases were essential for the successful transformation and sustainability of the culture of care, but we did not know at the beginning all that would be required or some of the challenges we would encounter. We learned as we went and adapted as we learned. Our experience clearly exemplified how proactive design meets real-world life. The key to our progress was responding to challenges as they unfolded and collaborating with faculty, staff, and students engaged in the change process. What follows is a high-level overview of Chamberlain's experiences and learning within each of the important phases of cultural transformation. Specific tools and examples of the application of *Chamberlain Care* for faculty and students are provided in Chapters 3 and 4.

Phase 1: It Starts at the Top

Culture is not delegable. The leader(s) must "own" culture, setting the vision and creating a compelling reason others should want to follow. What are our core values that are foundational to the culture we want to forge? What is possible? Why is it important? Why now? What will be required of me? This phase was among our most successful because we answered these questions effectively at the outset, which garnered support and engendered excitement among our colleagues for the potential of the initiative.

Kotter and Cohen (2002) considered the core problems people face when leading change. They interviewed 400 people from 130 organizations, concluding that the central issue was changing the behavior of people, and that successful change occurs when speaking to people's feelings. "People change what they do less because they are given *analysis* that shifts their *thinking* than because they are *shown* a truth that influences their *feelings*" (p. 1). This is especially true in large-scale changes (Kotter, 2012). In his book *Start With Why: How Great Leaders Inspire Everyone to Take Action,* Simon Sinuk (2011) urges leaders to share with employees the values and higher purpose of their organizations to help people feel connected and part of something bigger than themselves. When humans feel connected, trust is created and people feel inspired to act—not because they are paid to follow but because they want to.

Clearly articulating an organization's values, mission, and purpose provides employees clarity about how they should behave and helps them understand if and how their personal values align with the organization's values. Alignment of values creates an emotional connection between employees and the organization, which leads to employee loyalty. Bfau (2015) confirmed the power of mission and purpose and the impact they had on a transformation that took place at the large accounting firm KPMG. The goal of the initiative was to stir employees to take pride in their organization and work. Early in the process, the leaders used data to try to convince people, but it was only when the leaders abandoned their analytical approach and appealed to storytelling and emotion that people got excited and engaged in the project.

The Chamberlain experience was similar. Our compelling "reason why" stemmed from the powerful force of approximately 70,000 Chamberlain nurses (30,000 enrolled students and 40,000 alumni) and the impact they will have on patient care all over the world. We were inspired by the opportunity and the responsibility to graduate extraordinary nurses and understood that creating the right college culture for colleagues and students was the place to start. With an intentional effort, we knew that Chamberlain was more likely to develop a workforce of nurses who will have a positive impact on their work environments and a significant hand in transforming health care for the future.

Armed with a vision and reason why, we endeavored to gain buy-in from all Chamberlain leaders so that everyone was consistently communicating the same vision and goals. Our executive leadership team worked together to refine the vision and goals, and all committed to the journey, including being accountable to outcomes. The vision took shape around several themes:

1. There are 70,000 Chamberlain nurses in the world—let us do what we can to make those 70,000 extraordinary, with the potential to transform health care.

2. The way to graduate extraordinary nurses is to create an extraordinary environment—a caring environment where colleagues and students thrive—and to model behaviors exemplified by extraordinary nurses.

3. Let us create a culture that is vibrant and has purpose and meaning by actively honoring the students and colleagues we serve.

We understood from the beginning that it would take time to get total buy-in throughout the organization. We chose to start with the extended leadership team and a group of volunteer champions. Our idea was to develop a grassroots effort that would provide evidence of the powerful impact of care. We intended to produce results that would inspire others to follow, growing the initiative organically until the culture went viral.

The following are some of the strategies used to communicate the vision and gain buy-in from colleagues:

1. When the initiative first began, we organized a *Chamberlain Care* Steering Council comprised of the leadership team and volunteers from faculty, student services, admission, and other areas. We held a kickoff retreat for approximately 40 people at which we shared the vision, issued a challenge and call to action, set initial goals, and made assignments for implementation. In this way, we developed a group of "ambassadors" who committed to help drive the initiative.

2. In my role as the national president, I conduct "All Hands meetings" twice a year on every campus and with every team, including remote and home office colleagues. At the next series of meetings after the kickoff retreat, my presentation to team members included the vision, the why behind the vision and mission, a description of behaviors and beliefs that exemplify a caring

culture, and the initial goals for creating a culture of care focused on student success. The messages were repeated at all subsequent All Hands Meetings.

3. The *Chamberlain Care* Steering Council set goals and metrics and established a monthly meeting schedule to monitor progress of action plans and results.

4. We developed a scorecard to report to the college on the results of the initiative.

5. Because transformation is a team effort, we engaged in team-building exercises to create cohesive teams. We conducted several different workshops with groups of colleagues, presenting topics such as emotional intelligence, conflict management, goal setting, *Strength Finders,* and other tools for improving the leadership acumen and collaborative skills of team members. The workshops were designed to help leaders gain insight into how they could be more effective in their roles and to help identify those behaviors that might be getting in the way. Whether it is learning how to manage conflict better or helping to leverage the strengths of individuals on their team, the leaders walked away with tools that they could rely on to help increase their effectiveness.

Email from Charlotte campus president Catherine Holton to Ken Driscoll, senior director of human resources:

I just wanted to thank you for coming to the Charlotte campus last week to conduct the "How We Teach" training. The entire campus has been "buzzing" about it all week with increased energy and excitement toward our work and each other. I think it was just what we needed to increase our enthusiasm at a time when we were a little discouraged.

6. We learned early on that it was not enough for leaders to tell the stories about how care was making a difference in their work. We encouraged colleagues to tell their stories, as doing so was a way of demonstrating the embodiment of care and engaging us more as a community. This promotion of storytelling evoked a deep sense of ownership and pride in what we were creating—it became personal. When people started sharing care stories, the culture went viral.

There was skepticism at the beginning, especially among faculty, who are often suspicious of initiatives that feel like business projects without a higher purpose. However, it did not take long for faculty to see how a culture of care was empowering to them in their work with each other and with students. Faculty more than any others understand the impact to the student, the college, and society when a student is unsuccessful. When faculty began to trust that the initiative was about creating an environment where colleagues and students thrive, they began to adopt the language and behavior of the desired culture.

Of course, it is not enough to communicate the vision. People will watch to see what decisions leaders make and whether they truly live the values. When a leader does not live by the values, everything he or she is trying to accomplish is undermined. It was important for leaders at all levels to have self-awareness of the discrepancies between the values and vision they espoused and their actual behaviors as a leader. Leaders had to distinguish among their behaviors that actually enabled poor performance, those that failed to promote success where the potential existed, and those that truly engaged and empowered students and faculty to be successful.

Phase 2: Talking the Talk

Once a vision has been communicated, people need to know what it looks like, what it is, and what it is not. When the vision and goals were communicated to the college, we gave people the language of *Chamberlain Care* and asked them to use the language regularly. For example, it was suggested that admission advisors introduce prospective students to our philosophy of *Chamberlain Care* by telling them about our commitment to caring for students to help them succeed. At first, admission advisors found it awkward, but soon they were encouraged by the response from students and some began to adopt the language and philosophy. Whenever there was a site visit by an accreditor, we introduced our philosophy of *Chamberlain Care* and asked the site visitors to tell us whether they found evidence of the culture of care. Over time, the testimony of accreditation and regulatory visitors to the evidence of the care culture built confidence and a sense of pride among faculty and staff about our work.

From a Higher Learning Commission reaffirmation site visit report of evidence, 2015:

> P. 9, 1.B. The mission is articulated publicly.
>
> Based on conversations on the eight college campuses and follow-up conversations during the visit to the home office, the team concludes that Chamberlain's focus is on teaching-learning, and this commitment reflects its mission. Chamberlain Care is a distinguishing feature, and it is effectively communicated to students, healthcare partners, patients, and the greater community.

From a Higher Learning Commission campus evaluation visit report, Sacramento campus (10/11/2016):

> P. 6. Student and Faculty Resources and Support (Evidentiary Statements)
>
> Interviews with various personnel revealed that the staff are committed to effectively serving all students. Of particular note was the continued reference to the Chamberlain Care initiative during interviews with multiple groups conducted in accordance with this visit.

We found that the more people talked about *Chamberlain Care,* the more they began to believe it and behave it. Everyone in the college has annual performance objectives, which includes requiring everyone to demonstrate *Chamberlain Care* as it applies to their job. Team meetings began to include examples of delivering *Chamberlain Care* to colleagues or students.

From June Marlowe, vice president of student services:

> I have a bi-weekly meeting with my direct reports, and every meeting starts with a "Care Check-In." Knowing we only have an hour, there have been times that I've been tempted to skip this agenda item and move quickly to the work that needs to be done, but invariably I'm glad that I didn't. The stories shared by the team about care for self, for colleagues, and for students are incredibly motivating and often bring tears to my eyes. These stories are shared with the rest of the department in our monthly newsletter under the heading "Care Corner."

One notable strategy was the action of having a mortarboard in every meeting room to remind even those who did not have direct contact with students that the job of every person in the organization was to promote the graduation of our students and to recall that our deliberations should reflect their genuine concerns for a quality education.

In describing what *Chamberlain Care* meant, we defined *care* as "the excellent service we provide to each other and to our students to help students achieve their goals and reach their dreams." It meant service to support student success, not to do whatever it takes to make students happy. It was especially important to discuss with faculty what *Chamberlain Care* is not. At first, the faculty were the most resistant to the concept of "care for students." They were concerned that we expected faculty to give all students passing grades, or allow students special dispensation not to do the work assigned. One of the critical lessons we learned was the need to help sort out with faculty the difference between care for a student based on an understanding and appreciation of his or her capabilities as opposed to doing anything and everything to rescue a student who is unsuccessful. We needed to actively clarify what we meant by *care*. Care meant that faculty do not tell students who have a question to "look it up" without understanding whether the student made an effort to research an issue. Care meant helping students learn, which sometimes means providing extra assistance to a student who needs it. Care did not mean passing all students with an A. Care did not mean that all students would succeed, regardless of their effort. Care did not mean students were always right. One strategy that was successful with faculty was posing scenarios and asking faculty to describe caring approaches. In this way, we could identify misunderstandings and provide clarification. Once faculty understood that the expectation is that students will be held to a high standard—it is more about the way we do things than what we do that is most important—they were enthusiastic participants and supporters.

Anonymous faculty comments obtained from the annual employee engagement survey:

> I love making a difference for my students, who are typically from underrepresented groups in the U.S. I also am consistently impressed with the commitment to integrity at Chamberlain.

> Working with the team I work with has been the highlight of my professional career. The variation in talents and the like-minded determination in making our area the best at what we do makes an amazing combination.

> This organization (and my leaders) has always treated me with respect and recognized my work and successes. I have worked here since 2009 and I can honestly say this is the best job and group I have ever worked with, and I have worked for 40 years! The "honeymoon" phase hasn't ended, because everyone treats me with [same] genuine care and respect as the first day I started! I love my job!

> My fellow colleagues care about the students. They dedicate their whole being into mentoring and seeing students become successful, safe, practicing nurses. I like seeing the dedication in not only myself but my support staff around me.

> The reason for my high rating is the culture of Chamberlain Care, making a difference in students' lives, and supporting team members to achieve personal and professional goals.

> A culture of caring permeates my college. I feel that my professional growth is valued in my college.

> ➤ I have never ever worked in a place that truly is kind like this. My leaders are absolutely fabulous and support their team. It is an absolute honor to work in this team. I hope to have this job absolutely forever. Each team member is kind, respectful, and supportive your entire time. The leadership team and my colleagues reflect Chamberlain Care every single day.

> ➤ I appreciate the organizational commitment to supporting student success. Chamberlain Care has been further defined this past year and it is truly evident as being a part of our organizational culture/our DNA—it describes who we are and what we are all about—caring for and supporting the success of our students (and academic excellence). It has truly been effectively encultured throughout our organization. It is a thing!

> ➤ The culture on this campus is one of the BEST that I have been a part of in my 22 years in nursing. This is like my second family. I really appreciate my colleagues and our leadership.

Phase 3: Walking the Walk: Operationalizing the Model

Watson (2009) asserted that care must be operationalized in concrete acts if it is to be realized as care. To operationalize *Chamberlain Care,* we developed a framework that guides specific actions and specifies metrics used to measure our success. The framework is designed around phases in the student life cycle where we can make an impact on student success (Figure 2.1).

This framework was printed on tent cards for every colleague's desk as a reminder of our intentional culture of care and the opportunities where we can make a difference in our interaction with students. The framework includes measures of *care for colleagues* and addresses *care for students* throughout the student life cycle, beginning when a student applies and ending when the graduate is employed or returns to school for more education. We began with a focus on retention and created a pilot to test concepts.

Chamberlain's prelicensure BSN curriculum is organized in nine 16-week semesters, with each semester comprised of two 8-week sessions (a total of 18 sessions). Courses are 8 weeks in length. Many students transfer general education credits taken at other colleges and universities, so program lengths vary and some students start nursing courses earlier than others as a result. As a single-purpose nursing college, Chamberlain's curriculum included all required general education courses, which were dispersed throughout the curriculum.

In spring 2012, Chamberlain leaders analyzed aggregate student cohort retention from the July 2010 cohort, which showed that 28 percent of students were lost in the first five semesters (10 sessions). It is rare for students to be academically dismissed in the first two sessions of the program, although some students get into trouble early, which could encourage them to leave. Most leave school during the first two sessions for reasons unrelated to academics. Reasons given among students in the sample study were most often related to financial challenges, but other reasons were grades, family problems, change of career choice, and health problems. As a result of these findings, we focused the initial pilot of our initiative on the first nursing course of the program, believing that if we could improve retention early in the program, it would translate to improved graduation rates over time.

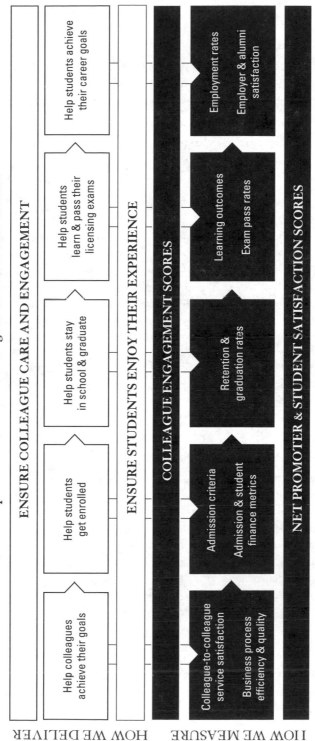

FIGURE 2.1 Operationalizing the *Chamberlain Care* Model.

A series of meetings was scheduled for sharing the vision of *Chamberlain Care* and the specifics of the pilot:

▸ A leadership kickoff workshop was held on February 13, 2012, to introduce *Chamberlain Care* and the pilot.

▸ A pilot project team kickoff workshop was held April 9 and 10, 2012.

▸ The pilot was launched for the first nursing course at two campuses in July 2012.

▸ Statistically significant results were observed from the July pilot; the pilot was expanded to two other campuses in March 2013.

▸ The pilot initiative was expanded to all campuses in September 2013.

▸ Based on the success of the pilot, several task forces were established to expand the impact.

The pilot is discussed in detail in Chapter 4, including a discussion of results from the pilot and ongoing work on retention.

Continuous process improvement. Courses are only one aspect of how we interact with students, albeit a critical one. Culture change must be supported with efficient and effective processes, which Chamberlain addressed through multiple quality improvement initiatives, including review of admission criteria success factors, revising the student open house to create a more engaging prospective student experience, initiatives to promote excellence in classroom instruction, a process for identifying and supporting high-risk students, and measures to improve postlicensure online student retention and satisfaction. Six to eight goals are established each year by the *Chamberlain Care* Steering Council to expand the focus and impact on retention and *Chamberlain Care.* The goals are integrated into individual leader performance goals to hold the team accountable for making progress.

Anonymous student comments obtained from a student survey:

Tinley Park, IL: Chamberlain displays its care in multiple ways. They provide many resources and much support. The staff actually care about my success. Having the NCLEX review and personal coaches keep me focused and on task.

Arlington, VA: I am thankful for Chamberlain College of Nursing for giving me all the resources to be a successful student and an extraordinary nurse in the future.

Columbus, OH: I am thankful to be at a school that genuinely cares for my success.

Chicago, IL: I can't believe that Chamberlain is investing this much into our success. I knew when I started this program that it was different. I know I can be successful. Thank you, Chamberlain. I can't wait to be that extraordinary nurse.

Phase 4: Inspecting What You Expect

The cultural transformation initiative was essentially a quality improvement project; therefore, impact had to be measured, results evaluated, and learning applied. Every goal we set and project we implemented as part of the cultural transformation initiative had metrics tied to it, and we reported regularly on those metrics to the entire College. The goals and metrics have been integrated into the college's systematic evaluation plan. To this day, 7 years after beginning the process, Chamberlain continues to establish annual

---

BOX 2.1

Examples of Key Metrics Tracked for Prelicensure and Postlicensure Programs

Key Performance Outcomes
- Student performance on national board examinations (i.e., NCLEX-RN, AANP or ANCC certifications)
- Retention and persistence
- Student results on standardized tests
- Program completion rates
- Evaluation of faculty's Master Instruction skills/behaviors
- Student and alumni's willingness to recommend their programs

Course Evaluation
- Student course and instructor satisfaction
- Student engagement
- Student's perception of care from faculty
- Course pass rates
- Course student/faculty ratios

Program Evaluation
- Alumni satisfaction with programs
- Alumni's application of knowledge, skills, and abilities learned
- Employer satisfaction with alumni preparation
- Employment rates
- Faculty engagement

---

goals for *Chamberlain Care,* and to publish a *Chamberlain Care* scorecard every semester to track the results, including retention after each semester, graduation rate, NCLEX-RN first-time pass rate, student satisfaction, and colleague engagement, to name a few. The *Chamberlain Care* Steering Council now meets quarterly instead of monthly. At quarterly meetings, the scorecard and progress on initiatives are reported on and reviewed. Box 2.1 provides the list of metrics tracked on the quarterly scorecard.

The results of initiatives are shared with the entire college during the National President's All Hands meetings twice a year. In this way, we hold ourselves accountable for delivering tangible results and benefit for the effort. These meetings also provide an opportunity to hear directly from the participants in all areas of the college the successes and challenges encountered in the cultural transformation. Learnings from these meetings provide guidance in revising implementation strategies to gain the greatest success.

Phase 5: Building the Foundation: Infrastructure to Support Culture

Because it is difficult, if not impossible, to train people to care, we are intentional about hiring caring people and providing them the appropriate training, support, and tools. We promote our *Chamberlain Care* culture in our recruiting advertising and make it an important part of interviews and screening.

From Dawn M. Gubanc-Anderson, DNP, MSN, RN, NE-A, BC, FACHE, associate professor, Cleveland campus:

As a nurse executive, I have always been keenly aware of the importance of culture in an organization. Culture impacts motivation, potential, and the art of possibility. As an employee, you know if your organization has a positive culture. You feel it in your being. You feel invigorated, appreciated, and recognized for the strengths you bring to [the] team.

I felt the positive culture immediately when I interviewed for my position at Chamberlain. It was the deciding factor in my decision to join the Chamberlain team. This transformative culture empowers me to bring the best learning environment to my students. It is the way we create extraordinary students. It is the Chamberlain difference! My students routinely comment on the amazing culture we create in the classroom.

Thank you for the opportunity to serve our students and fellow faculty members, Susan. It is a source of great professional joy and honor for me.

From Tamara Juanell Jones, MSN, RN, assistant professor, Charlotte campus:

As a student at Chamberlain, I experienced the caring and supportive culture of Chamberlain College of Nursing. Now that I am a nurse educator at Chamberlain, I am experiencing Chamberlain Care from a different perspective.

The moment I walked in the door for my interview on the Charlotte Chamberlain Campus, I felt the energy. I knew this was going to be the right place for me. The collegiality and teamwork amongst my colleagues is palpable. You can tell that everyone is on the same page: to ensure we care for our students and each other. The management team ensures this mindset continues through their transparency, approachability, and support. I have always said an organization will be strong if the leadership is strong. Furthermore, I truly feel valued and appreciated at Chamberlain, which is something that is truly important to me as an employee. This is also important for our students because that gives our students a positive impression of the college, the culture, and the education they are going to receive at Chamberlain. I am so proud to be a Chamberlain alumni and so honored to be a part of the Chamberlain team.

To enhance our ability to find the people who fit our culture of care, we collaborated with a third-party vendor to adapt our standard prehire assessment to evaluate caring behaviors in prospective colleagues. The prospective colleague's performance on the care scale is an important factor in hiring decisions.

Email from Student Support Advisor Tom Ryan to his supervisor, Sarah Nast:

I didn't really know what to expect when coming to Chamberlain, but I am so grateful that I said yes. You have been warm, welcoming, and have communicated that I am valuable to the team multiple times. Thank you for making me feel welcome here and for bringing a sense of CARE to the department. It has permeated our daily operations. Again, I appreciate you having me, and I'm grateful for every opportunity I've been given to shine and develop here.

From Kevin Letz, DNP, MBA, MSN, RN, CNE, CEN, FNP-C, ANP-BC, PCPNP-BC, FAANP, dean of academic operations and professor of the graduate program, family nurse practitioner track:

A culture of care in our area has had corollary benefits in both finding and retaining faculty. As we grow and faculty positions become open, we have a long list of interested parties wanting to be part of our team. I am constantly asked whether positions are open or will become open in the future. Additionally, we have had only one person leave our team over the years since our program track launched. Our comradery is evident to both those inside and outside our institution. Everyone wants to be part of the team who has fun at work and clearly respects one another. We celebrate team members' success and their special events and support one another through difficult times, whether work or personal in nature. A culture of care really resembles the creation of an extended family where members of your family become more important than any internal personal fulfillment. Our culture of care clearly adds to the engagement of our team and makes us want to come to work every day.

Culture fit is an important measure of performance and potential. Chamberlain colleagues are held accountable for the culture through their regular performance evaluations, which include a measure of whether they live and behave according to the college's TEACH values (teamwork, energy, accountability, community, heart). Our colleagues know that "how you do your job" is just as important as "what you do" in your job. For example, our value of "heart" requires people who respect each other and assume positive intent in colleagues. If we allow an employee to disrespect others, we undermine our culture and values.

We reinforce this standard during performance calibration sessions.

From Thomas Williams, vice president of marketing, who wrote about his revelation during one such session:

I knew our culture was taking hold when during performance review ratings of our direct reports, [the leader] recommended an "exceeds expectations" rating for one her directors. After presenting her rationale for the rating, she asked for feedback and learned from her colleagues that while the director had exceeded her annual goals, she had operated out of line with the values of Chamberlain Care and was consistently combative, noncollaborative, and unhelpful. The rating was lowered, and the manager used the feedback to coach the colleague. To everyone's delight, the colleague embraced and accepted the feedback, made changes to how she worked with others, and a year later was nominated for an award for living Chamberlain Care.

Another important practice in ensuring that a culture is sustainable is deliberately removing those who cannot or will not exemplify the culture. The true test of culture is whether the organization has the courage and fortitude to fire people who do not live the culture. Of course, this means that people need to understand and articulate the culture and the values underlying it if they are to be held accountable for them.

From Richard Cowling, former vice president of academic affairs:

We were in dire need of filling a critical position to lead one of our departments. The recruitment team identified an ideal candidate with the exact background, intelligence, and expertise in the field we sought. In spite of some vague misgivings about this candidate's communication style, we hired him almost immediately. Unfortunately, we learned within weeks of his hire that he was not a good fit for our culture. He was driven by a perception of being right at all costs, cared little for the opinions of others, dominated team meetings, and communicated passive-aggressively. He ended up being asked to leave the institution within 6 months of being hired. The negative outcomes of his short tenure were devastating to our institution: disillusionment of his team, delayed launch of strategic projects, damaged relationships with key institutional partners, and personal distress for him.

In addition to people, processes and technology can be important detractors or enhancers of culture. If a culture of care means that students receive prompt answers to queries about their classes, registration, financial aid, or other issues, then the management processes and technology must support the service intent and pledge. Opportunities for improvement remain for Chamberlain as we continue to evaluate what improvements we can make in the student experience.

From Sonya Evanosky, vice president of finance and strategy:

> Chamberlain's family nurse practitioner track grew rapidly due to student demand, but we learned that students were having difficulties finding practicum sites and preceptors. We realized we needed to provide a personal approach that was consistent with our culture of care. The approach we adopted involved practicum coordinators and support specialists proactively reaching out to students and checking on their progress in locating a preceptor and practicum site. Students were given coaching and encouragement, and those who continued to have difficulty were assigned a support specialist who helped the student develop his or her "elevator speech" or method for approaching preceptors and sites, and in some instances the specialist contacted sites directly on behalf of the student. We pursued this route because we thought it more clearly and directly demonstrated care than any of the other options, and students have responded favorably to this approach. One student posted to Facebook about her experience: "Pleasantly surprised! I just received a phone call from my practicum coordinator 'just to check in on me, see how I was doing, if there were any questions she could answer for me, or help me with anything at all.' Wow! She caught me totally off guard, but all my questions started popping into my head on cue. She even gave me her phone number with office hours. I feel so much better that I got to speak with someone directly (not just by email) and feel better informed about the practicum process now."

Phase 6: Built to Last

Prior to 2014, Chamberlain's cultural initiative was progressing with various pilots and projects to improve service and academic outcomes. By that time, every person had been introduced to the concepts and the goals. In 2014, Chamberlain took a big step in the enculturation process with the development of a *Chamberlain Care* enculturation workshop. A group of colleagues developed the workshop to drive home the values that we wanted exemplified in *Chamberlain Care*—care for self, care for colleagues, and care for students. We brought leaders from all areas of the organization to a training session, and through a "train the trainer" approach, the sessions were extended to the entire college.

The workshop was a day-long facilitated session that included several exercises to drive home the concepts important to the culture. The workshop was designed to help colleagues at all levels of the organization gain insight into what behaviors they were demonstrating that did or did not align with our desired culture of care and service. We defined what we meant by culture and why it mattered. The workshop created a common language of care building on our TEACH values and outlined a set of common behavioral expectations. It also helped participants gain a better understanding of themselves and how to work better with colleagues. It provided a framework for how we expected each other to act and a set of tools. Many commented that the tools they learned at the workshop helped them not only at work but also in their relationships outside of work and in their daily lives. After the workshop, every person got a care package with goodies and a copy of the tools that were introduced as a reminder of how to keep on track with the principles of care. All 1,200 colleagues went through the training, and it is now incorporated in Chamberlain's new colleague 2½-day orientation/enculturation training.

Of all we have done in our journey to develop a culture of care, the enculturation workshop may have had the biggest impact so far. The grassroots effort that had taken place over the preceding 2 years had laid the groundwork. The message and vision were not new. But when we brought people together to inspire and provide tools for success, the energy was contagious. The key was in giving all colleagues the same message at around the same time, as it created a critical mass of people who were inspired by the message and the goals—the culture of care went viral. Now everyone at Chamberlain understands what *Chamberlain Care* means to colleagues and students. It is a source of pride. Colleague comments after the workshop reflect some of what they learned:

From Courtney Fritts, senior executive advisor:

The workshop was about really trying to do the things to improve who you are and to recognize your strengths and how people see you and value you, and I think it was amazing.

From Jennifer Wood, instructor, Atlanta campus:

If you develop that culture that everybody is shining in their strengths and accepting of others' strengths, then the students are [going to] come in feeling that appreciation and that they matter and be invited to be in a place where they can develop their own career.

From Maria Jose Bassett, health care development specialist:

We call it care, but it's how do we take care of each other, how do we act with each other, how do we behave with each other.

From Trish Hughes, EdD, MSN, MBA, CRNP, former Arlington campus president, current director of postlicensure program regulation and accreditation:

As one of the original workshop facilitators when Chamberlain Care became a bedrock of our culture, I have to say that it was one of the most rewarding roles I've had. I faced colleagues at the beginning of those workshops who you could tell from body language thought this was all another bunch of fluff under a new name. Some of those colleagues are still with Chamberlain and are role models for Chamberlain Care. It is a testament to how transformative 'care' can be in a person's life. And those who are not still with Chamberlain? Well, that's a testament to how a strong culture of care will help those who cannot embrace it to move on to other places more comfortable to them.

The main message conveyed to colleagues at the workshop is that Chamberlain cares about them and wants them to love what they do. Colleagues were encouraged to "fill their cups" by caring for themselves so that they could bring their best selves to their jobs to do the important work of helping students achieve success. Many colleagues wrote emails to me afterward remarking that they have never felt so cared for and empowered by an employer. Their comments confirm that by caring for our colleagues, we give them the resources to care for students. The results show in our colleague engagement scores that are at world-class levels year after year (and that spiked up in 2014—the year we conducted the workshops; see Chapter 3).

CARE EXEMPLARS

In creating a culture of care, two key elements emerged from the work that have had a significant impact (Figure 2.2). These care exemplars are presented in Chapters 3 and 4:

> ▶ The first is *Master Instruction,* our philosophy of teaching excellence, presented in Chapter 3. *Master Instruction* defines how Chamberlain cares for its faculty as we support and develop our faculty. *Master Instruction* also exemplifies how Chamberlain cares for students by striving to deliver an outstanding student experience.

> ▶ The second is the *Chamberlain Care* Student Success Model, Chamberlain's program of supporting and helping prelicensure students succeed, presented in Chapter 4. The *Chamberlain Care* Student Success Model begins when a student

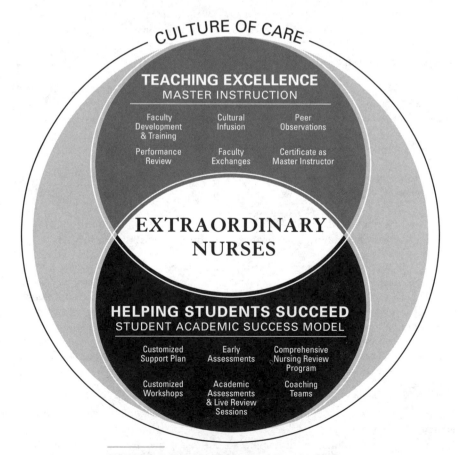

FIGURE 2.2 Three key elements of *Chamberlain Care*.

is admitted and extends through graduation until a student passes NCLEX-RN and is employed. Chapter 4 also provides examples of application of *Chamberlain Care* initiatives for postlicensure students.

"TO INFINITY AND BEYOND"

Cultural transformation is not a "one and done" initiative. We continue to be very intentional about all things culture. It must be central to all decisions, interactions with colleagues, partners, and students. We will continue to strive to make a caring culture part of our DNA, which includes celebrating successes, reinforcing the concepts, and rewarding the champions. We believe that we have created the kind of environment where people want to work—where they are doing important work, changing lives, and feeling supported and cared for themselves.

Our vision and ultimate aspirational goal is that by living *Chamberlain Care,* we graduate extraordinary nursing professionals who transform health care worldwide. How do we know our graduates are extraordinary? What exactly is an extraordinary nurse? In Chapter 5, we describe our current research initiatives to attempt to answer those very questions. In the meantime, we rely on feedback from our students and from health care partners to confirm that we are making progress toward the goal of preparing the kind of professionals they want to hire.

From Jenny Wolinski, OR manager of clinical practice, Advocate Lutheran General Hospital, Park Ridge, IL:

Chamberlain students are more focused, driven, and well prepared, and they have their act together more so than other schools of nursing students and new grads I've worked with. A Chamberlain student is in our OR residency program now, and we've had at least five to six other Chamberlain graduates in the OR [who] successfully went through our OR residency program, are still working here, and are working out very well!

From Jessica Cooper, Chamberlain Irving campus student:

My name is Jessica Cooper, and I am completing my last year at Chamberlain College of Nursing Irving Campus. A friend who heard the open house info on the radio station led me to this school. After applying to several different community colleges and being wait listed and not feeling confident, I decided to attend the open house. I had the best time there, I was being treated as a student who already attended, I got to experience the state-of-the-art Sim Lab that Chamberlain is known for, and at the point my decision was made. My admission process was smooth, from the welcome of the Campus President, the Dean of Instruction, to the advisors; I knew that they wanted me to be a part of the team. Now that I have completed a full year at Chamberlain with a determined plan to graduate next February, I can honestly say that this is the best decision that I have made. The class sizes are perfect, the teachers are committed to you succeeding, the Center for Academic Success has an unlimited amount of resources with a manager who holds a PhD. I have had the pleasure of attending various clinical sites, and they all remember Chamberlain students, so there is an opportunity for networking. Less than a year from now, BSN, RN will be at the end of my name, and I can't wait to become an Extraordinary Nurse.

From Malinda Lebrun, Chamberlain North Brunswick campus student:

It has truly been an honor and a blessing to be a student at Chamberlain. I am surrounded by great professors who not only care for me but always go out of their way to [ensure] that I am getting the best education. In addition, the tutoring and workshops that are offered through the CAS is a great help in helping me succeed in all my courses. At Chamberlain, extraordinary care, reverence, and professionalism is shown among both faculty and students. I am confident that I will be graduating as a proficient health care professional ready to have a positive impact in people's lives.

From Corey Mills, Charlotte campus student:

Chamberlain College of Nursing is truly a nursing school like no other. From the moment I heard about Chamberlain, I have had only positive experiences. I started at a different nursing program. I researched many nursing schools and looked at the different aspects of each program. A friend told me about a nursing school that was opening in Charlotte, NC. I then decided to research that school. That school happened to be Chamberlain College of Nursing. I read such positive reviews, and I saw only positive things about the school. I called to find out more information, and I attended an open house. From the moment I walked on the campus, I was welcomed like I was already family. The staff was so welcoming and answered any questions I had. I decided to apply, and I got accepted. I was so excited to begin this new journey at a nursing school that truly cares about their students. I moved to Charlotte, NC, and began orientation. I have seen firsthand how much the faculty, colleagues, and staff help the students and how they want each and every student to succeed. They know every student by name. I moved to a city knowing no one and have met so many friends through Chamberlain, and I can truly say that I have family at this school. This school inspires me to care for others and to become the extraordinary nurse that I know I can be. The resources Chamberlain provides and the staff they chose exhibit the Chamberlain Care Model, which is a caring environment. I applied for a work-study job in the SIMCare Center because I wanted to work for place that puts employees and students first and centers the job on caring for others. I am proud to work and study at Chamberlain College of Nursing, and I am excited to graduate in a year to become a Chamberlain nurse.

From Christina Rucker, Phoenix campus student:

As a new student at Chamberlain, I was assigned to a student mentor [who] was further ahead in the program to answer any questions I may have or just help me with this new endeavor I had started. I liked being able to ask a student questions and get answers from a student's perspective. As I progressed through the program, I became the student further along in the program, speaking to the new students and answering their questions they were afraid to ask the faculty.

Throughout my entire program, I have been supported by faculty and the resources that Chamberlain offers. I have always felt comfortable approaching faculty to ask for help if needed or wanted. The CAS has also been a helpful resource for me. I would attend scheduled reviews that were held for the class I was in, and sometimes I would have one-to-one meetings with a professional tutor to further my understanding of certain concepts.

Nursing is a second career for me, so as someone [who] is older than most students and has been out of school as long as I had been, I needed to choose a school that could be supportive for me, that offered resources outside of regular lecture. Nursing school is probably one of the toughest things I have ever done, but also one of the most rewarding things I've ever done in my life. Now that I am 1 week away from graduation, I can say I feel completely prepared for my upcoming career. I'm so glad I chose Chamberlain.

From Carolyn Ruud, DNP, RN, CCRN CVRN-BC SCRN, March 2017 DNP graduate:

Chamberlain Cares: My experience

Going back to school after many years as a nurse is challenging. As I worked, many of my nurse peers complimented me on the way that I shared information with new nurses and how well the nurses understood information I shared. I was smitten with the educator bug! I would always be assigned the students on the unit and the new graduates to precept. I took classes in sharing information and adult learning. I participated in shared governance and excelled in the development of implementation. I enjoyed this until one day one of my peers asked me why I did not go on to get my master's degree. I could not answer why except that we really couldn't afford a college bill, as we had been foster parents and our savings had been depleted.

I went to the cafeteria one day and saw the table set up for Chamberlain College of Nursing! I spoke with the recruiter, who assured me that we had great benefits at our hospital that will cover most of the program. Well there went my only barrier to going on with obtaining my master's degree! As I learned how to learn again, I met some of what I believe are the best instructors. I was pushed to find out new things about myself, supported always and to this day have some of the AHA moments saved in my "toolbox" as well as Impeccable APA formatting! OK, so now I was done! No more school, right? I could officially teach nurses, work at the bedside, and care for patients. My two most favorite reasons to go to work.

Being a bedside nurse is all I ever wanted to do. I liked research and solving bedside problems but am not a "researcher." Obtaining a PhD was not one of my interests. As far as I was concerned, I was done. Then I started reading about the DNP movement to provide leadership skills to nurses at the point of care! This sounded right for me. Really, going to school again? Was I really wanting to start this again? I called and spoke with the Chamberlain recruiter. Having been through the master's program, I was excited to learn new things but scared at the same time. I still struggled with some of the subjects and did not want to fail. I was reassured that support would be there for me along the way from the faculty to the librarians and the team. Knowing that this was a new program to Chamberlain, I was expecting some challenges but felt they would be handled well. The program challenged me to find out things about myself I did not know or have the confidence in knowing. I found out I understood process improvement and could add value to any team I am asked to be a part of. When I was struggling, it was really great to be able to reach out to the leadership team to guide and support me. There were helpful webinars, such as writing success and [a] project and practicum Q&A forum. These helped support my weak areas and [gave] me tools for success. Just as I was completing my DNP project, it was pulled from the institution because of a computer upgrade. I was sure I would have to delay graduation for one or two sessions. I was very down. Luckily it was spring break, and I spoke with my faculty and was able to come up with a plan. Given the opportunity to still succeed was essential. I was supported in my project, supported in revising my final document over the next few weeks. The faculty and leadership of the DNP program are the best. I was given every opportunity to develop a DNP plan that fit my needs and challenges. Had I not had the support of all the faculty or been in a traditional program, I think I would have been encouraged to postpone. Through this support and planning, my project was completed and I graduated on time. I am proud to be a Chamberlain graduate!

From Tracey Moffatt, RN, BSN, MHA, system chief nursing officer and senior vice president of quality, Ochsner Health System:

Nurses don't touch one life or 10 lives or even 1,000 lives in their careers. Through care delivered with their own hands, they may touch tens of thousands of lives over the course of their career. As important as it is to care compassionately for patients and their families, the new nurses they influence during their careers can have an even greater impact.

Hiring a new nurse is one of our most important functions in nursing leadership. But the process of hiring is only the beginning. Instilling the right behaviors, setting the right tone, and modeling compassion is where our influence as nurse leaders lies. As a health system, Ochsner hosts hundreds of nursing students every year. And, frankly, I believe that is an opportunity to influence young professionals the first time they step foot into a clinical setting. It's something Ochsner Health System invests in. And we cherish the opportunity to do so.

The Ochsner Health System is thrilled to join with Chamberlain College of Nursing through our unique partnership and share in bringing the opportunity for more people to pursue the nursing profession. Hospitals working closely with academic institutions of Chamberlain's caliber is vital to supporting the continued growth of professional nursing.

References

Adtalem Global Education Human Resources Data System, 2017. Downers Grove, IL.

American Association of Colleges of Nursing. (2016). Fact sheet: Enhancing diversity in the workforce. Retrieved June 25, 2017, from http://www.aacn.nche.edu/media-relations/fact-sheets/enhancing-diversity

Bfau, B. N. (2015). How an accounting firm convinced its employees they could change the world. *Harvard Business Review.* Retrieved June 25, 2017, from https://hbr.org/2015/10/how-an-accounting-firm-convinced-its-employees-they-could-change-the-world

Kenny, B. (2007). The coming crisis in employee turnover. *Forbes.* Retrieved June 25, 2017, from https://www.forbes.com/2007/04/24/employees-turnover-careers-lead-careers-cz_bk_0425turnover.html

Kotter, J. P. (2012). *Leading change.* Boston: Harvard Business Review Press.

Kotter, J. P., & Cohen, D. S. (2002). *The heart of change: Real-life stories of how people change their organizations.* Boston: Harvard Business Review Press.

Sinuk, S. (2011). *Start with why: How great leaders inspire everyone to take action.* New York: Penguin.

Watson, J. (2009). *Assessing and measuring caring in nursing and healthcare.* New York: Springer.

3

Promoting Teaching Excellence:
A Culture of Care for Faculty

Candice Phillips, PhD, RN, APRN, CNM, CNE
Laura Fillmore, DNP, MSN, RN, CNE
Chad O'Lynn, PhD, RN, CNE, ANEF
Kellie Bassell, EdD, MSN, RN, CNE
Linda Hollinger-Smith, PhD, RN, FAAN, ANEF

A CULTURE OF CARE FOR FACULTY

Change is difficult, both to implement and to sustain. An organization will likely return to its "norm" or previous state unless a shared responsibility for implementing and sustaining the initiative is created (Sabelli & Dede, 2013). Uniting colleagues in a collaborative vision of *Chamberlain Care* through the enculturation workshops inspired college-wide enthusiasm for the values required to improve service and academic outcomes. Integral to our shift from a traditional academic organization to a more caring, service-oriented one was an intentional focus on improvement of teaching practice through the integration of *Master Instruction,* Chamberlain's approach to teaching excellence. This emphasis on teaching excellence provided faculty effective teaching and learning strategies to support student success while establishing tangible goals and expectations of care behaviors relevant to the faculty role. Through *Master Instruction,* faculty were empowered with skills and resources to meet our service intent to care for students and help them reach their educational goals and dreams.

CARE EXEMPLAR: *MASTER INSTRUCTION*

For many years, nurse academicians and other leaders in higher education have called for a paradigm shift in the way educators view the teaching and learning process (Bain, 2004; Bass, 2012; Benner, Sutphen, Leonard, & Day, 2010; National Research Council, 2000). Methods from past experience and education can no longer be used to meet present and future students' educational needs. New ways of teaching are required to graduate nurses who think critically while caring for diverse populations in a changing health care landscape (Benner et al., 2010; Sherwood & Horton-Deutsch, 2015). Our aim to promote teaching excellence in a culture of care aligned with wider intentioned efforts to improve teaching and learning in higher education.

This impetus for change led us to revise the first nursing course in the curriculum. This course was selected as a pilot by the *Chamberlain Care* Steering Council, a group of leaders and innovative faculty who assembled to discuss strategies for implementing learning-centered teaching. These discussions about how to improve teaching practice led to Ken Bain's (2004) landmark work, *What the Best College Teachers Do,* in which he describes how an authentic learning environment both challenges and supports students as they apply complex concepts to real-life situations. Bain's premise that the best faculty members "help their students learn in ways that make a sustained, substantial, and positive influence on how students think, act, and feel" (2004, p. 5) provided the perfect platform for teaching excellence in a culture of care. From this principle, Chamberlain's pedagogy, called *Master Instruction,* was conceived.

Master Instruction Philosophy and Pedagogy

Master Instruction is a philosophy and an attitude exemplified in interactions with students that supports them in developing new learning strategies and gaining deep learning. Through *Master Instruction,* faculty use pedagogical approaches beyond traditional content-based lectures to facilitate student learning of new competencies while creating an active learning environment that is aligned with the realities of today's nursing practice. *Master Instruction* places emphasis on transformational teaching and learning, and includes the purposeful use of instructional methods such as active, student-centered, collaborative, experimental, and problem-based learning, among others. The pedagogy of *Master Instruction* aligns with *Chamberlain Care,* equipping faculty to accompany students on their journey of learning, caring for and about them, and bringing learning to life. Understanding how students learn and assessing and meeting individual learning styles and needs are important to engage students effectively in developing successful nursing practice (Felver et al., 2010). Also important is helping faculty develop skill in aligning instructional strategies with learning outcomes and integrating current knowledge, trends, and technology advances into education (Forneris & Fey, 2016). The pedagogy of *Master Instruction* assists faculty in developing competencies needed to influence student success while supporting faculty collaboration and inquiry and contributing to the scholarship of nursing and nursing education. The most critical aim of *Master Instruction* is that it facilitates development of faculty competency across the career trajectory, providing tools to do the important work of helping students achieve success.

Master Instruction Implementation

Implementing the pedagogy of *Master Instruction* involved many steps. *Master Instruction* was introduced in the first nursing course during the pilot in 2012. After the perceived success of the pilot, *Master Instruction* was rolled out across the college to further cultural transformation through teaching excellence. A small evaluation study conducted shortly after the *Master Instruction* pilot used student and faculty focus groups to gather general feedback on *Master Instruction* implementation and perceived outcomes. Initial findings suggested increased satisfaction among students and faculty, and faculty reported a sense of validation of their roles as educators and transformation of their teaching behaviors. Rollout included three key action steps: establishment of a faculty development team to help faculty transition from their current methods of teaching to using the learning-centered approach of *Master Instruction,* appointment of *Master Instruction* champions to assist faculty developers in implementing *Master Instruction,* and the initiation of the *Master Instruction* peer observation process. Details regarding the outcomes of the application of *Master Instruction* and the observation process are discussed later in the chapter.

Faculty Development: Leading Teaching Excellence Through Master Instruction

Efforts to support and guide faculty development—particularly in a changing environment—are critically important for advancing scholarly competence (Sarikaya, Kalaca, Yegen, & Cali, 2010). In 2013, Chamberlain created the Center for Faculty Excellence (CFE) to improve the teaching skills of faculty, increase academic effectiveness, and advance the intentional effort of culture change. The CFE is a centralized yet geographically distributed national team consisting of the dean of faculty, four faculty development specialists, a senior instructional designer, and a web designer, who provide resources to guide and support development of beginning and experienced educators at Chamberlain. Our faculty development specialists strategized with faculty and leaders to formulate an efficient plan to implement *Master Instruction* while developing resources to enhance the effectiveness of faculty and the learning experience of students. Jasimuddin and Hasan (2015) point out that a supportive culture is vital to systemic educational improvements. Through strategic faculty development, Chamberlain supported faculty to develop their identity as excellent nurse educators by helping them internalize new beliefs, values, and attitudes toward teaching. Explicitly promoting teaching excellence through *Master Instruction* has had a positive and sustained impact on individual and collective teaching practices, as well as on student outcomes (see Outcomes of *Master Instruction* section). This transformation of both faculty member and student represents a shift from the traditional faculty-centered approach that has driven the delivery of educational content in academia toward a student-centered approach to learning that guides students to seek and apply knowledge in new ways to develop critical thinking and problem-solving skills (Schaefer & Zygmont, 2003).

Master Instruction *Champions: Agents of Change*

With a vast cadre of full- and part-time faculty distributed among 20 campuses and online programs across the country, change management is complex. To facilitate the use of *Master Instruction,* champions were utilized as change agents. As evidenced in nursing literature, champions are highly effective as agents of change in promoting positive outcomes through focused commitment and strong motivation, which can lead to sustainable transformation (Banks et al., 2014; Grealish, Henderson, Quero, Phillips, & Surawski, 2015; Jornsay & Garnett, 2014; Kaasalainen et al., 2015; Mount & Anderson, 2015). Our faculty development specialists recruited enthusiastic faculty and leaders to serve as champions to assist in the college-wide transformation of teaching practice through *Master Instruction.*

Working alongside faculty developers, *Master Instruction* champions generated trust, energy, insight, and commitment necessary for faculty to embrace the instructional expectations of *Master Instruction.* Paradeise and Thoenig (2013) contend that collaboration between and among faculty developers, champions, and faculty, along with implementation of appropriate teaching methodologies and resources, enhances the efficiency and performance of faculty while improving faculty work satisfaction and teaching confidence.

Initially, *Master Instruction* champions attended an intimate roundtable discussion to learn about our new learning-centered pedagogy. They also had the opportunity to explore an electronic graphic novel that adapted the symbolic contents of a well-known story, guiding them on a journey of reflection to transform teaching practice. Following the initial roundtable discussion, regular and ongoing virtual meetings were conducted to support and sustain the engagement of *Master Instruction* champions. These meetings serve as a venue to openly celebrate successes, share struggles, and gain encouragement, support, and feedback to advance *Master Instruction.* Additional *Master Instruction* teaching strategies (text based, audio, and video) are presented for others to incorporate.

According to Rogers (2010), interpersonal communication and social structures are critical contributors in the successful diffusion of innovation. Through continuing support and provision of faculty development resources, and through the dedicated efforts of our champions, *Master Instruction* is now flourishing at the national and location/ program levels and advancing our commitment to build a caring culture of teaching excellence (see Outcomes of *Master Instruction*).

Master Instruction *Observation: Peer Review of Teaching*

Master Instruction supports faculty practice, growth, and development in six broad areas: content management, active learning, relevance, facilitation, integration, and learning environment. These characteristics of *Master Instruction* are the performance criteria on which our observation process is based (see the *Master Instruction* Classroom Observation form in Appendix A). The *Master Instruction* observation process was developed to improve teaching practice and enhance student learning experiences and outcomes. This formative peer review process includes self- and dialogic reflection to expand faculty perspectives in identifying strengths and opportunities for improvement in their teaching practices

Brett, Branstetter, and Wagner (2014) proposed that respect, support, feeling valued, and trust/teamwork are key elements of a caring climate that support successful peer review. These caring qualities underpin our observation process, along with mutual trust and collaboration between participants. Emphasis in our review of teaching is placed on faculty growth and development to advance teaching practice, not on formal evaluation of performance. Our belief is that peer observation, conducted in a supportive environment, fosters reflection, self-awareness, and personal growth and development as an educator. Quality teaching is integral to a culture of care and service, and peer observation that supports growth in teaching and learning is central to enhanced teaching practice.

Chamberlain utilizes three phases of observation to provide faculty opportunity to examine their teaching practices and deepen their understanding of qualities in need of improvement (Kopelman & Vayndorf, 2012). Prior to the observation, the designated observer reviews the self-reflection of the faculty member being observed, then meets with the faculty member to discuss his or her teaching goals. During the observation, a Likert scale is used to record responses of each characteristic of *Master Instruction* demonstrated, as well as constructive, content-rich feedback to promote personal and professional development. Following the observation, the observer shares his or her insights from the review with the faculty colleague in a private meeting. The purpose of this meeting is to expand perspectives through dialogic reflection to transform teaching practice. According to Atkinson and Bolt (2010), the collegiality developed through shared experiences provides opportunity to communicate with colleagues, enjoy fellowship, and benefit from each other's knowledge and experience. At Chamberlain, our goal is for peer-supported review of teaching to forge a shared perception of quality outcomes and commitment to advance standards of excellence in teaching. Two seasoned faculty members from our MSN program remarked how the *Master Instruction* observation process led to collaborative reflection, professional learning conversations, and improvement-directed practice. Both the observer and observee commented that the review process was stimulating and encouraging, and it empowered them to improve their work as educators. Early outcomes from our *Master Instruction* observation process are reported later in the chapter.

Master Instructor Distinction

To distinguish faculty who strive for excellence in teaching, the award of Master Instructor distinction was established. At the heart of this distinction is *Master Instruction* and *Chamberlain Care* as the essence of teaching excellence. Distinction requirements are both academic and professional, and include selected professional development courses, peer observation, self-reflection, scholarly dissemination, and national nursing academic standards. Faculty who earn the Master Instructor distinction are awarded college lapel pins and email badges to signify their dedication to teaching excellence. Master Instructors are supported by faculty development specialists to provide academic coaching and formal mentoring to new and continuing faculty across the organization.

Master Instruction Resources: Teaching Excellence Comprehensive Program

Central to advancing teaching excellence was the provision of a comprehensive new faculty success program. A structured faculty development plan, titled the *Teaching Excellence Comprehensive Program,* was developed to transition new faculty across their first year of teaching at Chamberlain through the instructional expectations of *Master Instruction.* Included in the program are Teaching Excellence Foundations, an overview of skills and resources required for the academic role; Teaching Excellence Concepts, an eRepository of eLearning interactives that address key topics for faculty teaching and development; and Teaching Excellence Curriculum, an index of required

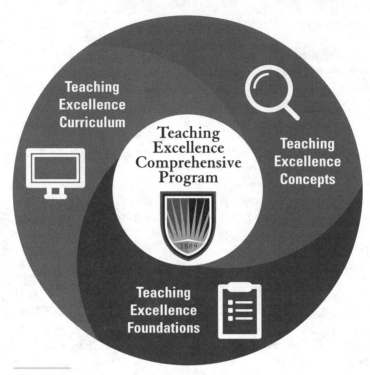

FIGURE 3.1 The Teaching Excellence Comprehensive Program.

and recommended faculty development courses and resources (Figure 3.1). According to Halstead (2007), new nurse educators must shift emphasis from delivery of quality patient care to delivery of quality student education, acquiring needed teaching competencies foundational to fulfillment of the academic role. The Teaching Excellence Comprehensive Program guides new faculty in the development of competencies specific to education through the pedagogical base of *Master Instruction* that integrates the art and science of nursing practice with the teaching and learning process.

Teaching Excellence Foundations: Onboarding Resource

Integral to the successful onboarding of new faculty is familiarization with organizational resources. As a focused checklist of skills and resources essential to teaching preparedness, Teaching Excellence Foundations ensures consistency in training of new faculty across the organization. At Chamberlain, we aim to recruit and retain best-in-class faculty who embody caring behaviors and attributes of teaching excellence. Nursing literature tells us that faculty who enter the academic setting from clinical practice are often surprised at the informality of the orientation process (Peters & Boylston, 2006; Roberts, Chrisman, & Flowers, 2013). Orientation to the role must be addressed to ensure quality education for students and rewarding work experiences for faculty (Schoening, 2013). Our belief is that faculty who receive early supportive orientation to the organization will be well prepared to provide exceptional experiences to students, resulting in superior academic outcomes and continuing commitment to the academic institution.

Within the first 30 days of hire, faculty are introduced to the systems and applications required for new faculty, specific policies and processes outlined by human resources, and expectations delineated in our academic handbooks. Also introduced at this time are the fundamental processes related to teaching preparedness, which includes the opportunity to observe seasoned faculty members to gain insight into *Master Instruction* pedagogy. Providing new faculty with the opportunity to observe classes conducted by different faculty and including all aspects of learning not only exposes them to the use of *Master Instruction* but also allows them to analyze different teaching styles that they might emulate in their own learning environments.

The Teaching Excellence Foundations checklist is also used by academic leaders as a review of resources for existing faculty. New resources are continually available at the college, and the use of this source ensures that all faculty are introduced to important resources in a timely fashion. A companion facilitators' guide for academic leaders provides guidelines for the use of the Teaching Excellence Foundations resource in establishing regular and ongoing discussions with new faculty to guide and support their successful transition to the college. Many colleagues expressed appreciation for the provision of these resources through emails or survey comments, stating that the resources empowered them to lead teaching excellence and support their team to be even more successful. Their comments confirm that caring for our colleagues by ensuring their success gives them the resources they need to care for students.

Teaching Excellence Concepts

Vyas, Faith, Selvakumar, Pulimood, and Lee (2016) point out that "just-in-time" eLearning can enhance educational reform. A repository of eLearning interactives, called *Teaching Excellence Concepts,* was developed to address key topics in faculty development and to support faculty learning preferences. These learning activities are thematically aligned to structure and sequence learning, and address academic alignment, academic integrity, grading and scholarship essentials, clinical teaching, distinct attributes of the college, and *Master Instruction.* These activities also serve as key learning components in the Teaching Excellence Curriculum (discussed later).

Faculty can use the Teaching Excellence Concepts eRepository to personalize learning, taking into account their experience, knowledge, and learning goals. Faculty leaders can use these learning activities to facilitate live or virtual, individual and/or collective discussions to advance teaching competencies. Learning activities in one topic area can be completed for an in-depth exploration of essential content, or individual activities can be completed to customize the learning experience based on learning style, special needs, or level of competency. In this way, the Teaching Excellence Concepts eRepository promotes varied opportunities for meeting individual, team, and program learning needs. Faculty and leaders comment regularly that the Teaching Excellence Concepts are helpful, practical, relevant, and engaging. The many uses of this eRepository make them a "go-to" resource for faculty on a regular basis.

Teaching Excellence Curriculum

Higher education literature tells us that an organization's commitment to excellence in teaching is a primary driver of faculty satisfaction (Candela, Gutierrez, & Keating, 2015; Steinert et al., 2016) and of student satisfaction and success (Ardisson, Smallheer, Moore, & Christenbery, 2015; Merillat & Scheibmeir, 2016; Witte & Jansen, 2016). The Teaching Excellence Curriculum, which includes required and recommended courses and resources to transition new faculty across their first year of teaching, was developed to promote satisfaction in the educator role and recruitment and retention of highly performing faculty to the institution, while delivering on our commitment to student success and satisfaction.

Required courses within the Teaching Excellence Curriculum are logically sequenced (Box 3.1) and use scaffolding strategies to move faculty progressively toward stronger understanding and, ultimately, greater skill in the teaching and learning process (Box 3.2). Required courses within the curriculum culminate in Master Instructor Level 1 distinction.

BOX 3.1

Teaching Excellence Curriculum Course Descriptions

CCN-101: Essential Guide for New Faculty Success

This course introduces faculty to the nurse educator role at Chamberlain University College of Nursing. Emphasis is placed on distinct attributes of the college, including *Chamberlain Care®* and *Master Instruction* pedagogy. The course presents an overview of the Learning Studio, Chamberlain curricula, policies, and evaluation processes to promote successful transitioning. This course presents professional development of faculty by enhancing skills, knowledge, and attitudes to facilitate student learning utilizing *Master Instruction.*

CCN-102: Essential Guide for Clinical Faculty Success

This course transitions new clinical faculty to the clinical nurse educator role, and enhances professional development for both beginning and experienced nurse educators by instilling competencies necessary for effective clinical education and nurturing greater fulfillment in the academic role. From pre- and post-conference planning to student evaluation and *Master Instruction* strategies in the clinical setting, each FACET offers innovative, instructional activities relevant to clinicians-turned-academic-educator. Essential resources provide integral support for real-world experiences.

CCN-110: *Master Instruction:* Chamberlain Care in Action

This course introduces the pedagogy of *Master Instruction* as *Chamberlain Care* in Action. Faculty venture into a transformative learning experience that models how transformative learning occurs. Through accessing and receiving the symbolic contents of a well-known story, and by analyzing its underlying premises, faculty are guided to ask questions and challenge assumptions as they reflect upon and develop insight into their teaching practice. This course can be used among faculty teams to bring ideas and insight to a collective process of reflection to generate shared meanings.

CCN-115: *Master Instruction:* Evidence-Based Teaching

The course presents an overview of three learning theories: Behaviorism, Cognitivism, and Constructivism. Faculty are guided to develop a deeper understanding of transformational teaching and learning with an emphasis on active learning, student-centered learning collaborative learning, experimental learning and problem-based learning. This course supports professional development of faculty by enhancing skills, knowledge, and attitudes to engage students in their classrooms utilizing *Master Instruction.*

BOX 3.1

Teaching Excellence Curriculum Course Descriptions (*Continued*)

CCN-120: Essential Guide for Scholarship

This course introduces faculty to the full range of scholarship within Chamberlain University College of Nursing. Emphasis is placed on the relevance and value of Boyer's Model of Scholarship to the unique culture of Chamberlain. Defining characteristics of the four standards of scholarship are highlighted: discovery, teaching, application in nursing practice, and integration of ideas from nursing and other disciplines. These standards of scholarship are examined as they are used to guide academic rank advancement. eLearning interactivities provide opportunity for application and synthesis of essential content, as well as deep reflection. This course supports professional development of faculty by enhancing skills, knowledge, and attitudes to expand the scope of recognized scholarly activities, guide individual career planning, and demonstrate the growth of the profession over time.

CCN-130: Essential Guide for Advancing Faculty Success

This course expands upon CCN-101: Essential Guide for New Faculty Success to advance new faculty performance in the nurse educator role at Chamberlain University College of Nursing. Emphasis is placed on teaching best practices to ensure student success, including grading essentials, discussion standards, and strategies to promote academic integrity and manage student performance issues. eLearning interactivities provide opportunity for application and synthesis of essential content, as well as deep reflection. This course supports professional development of faculty by enhancing skills, knowledge, and attitudes to facilitate student learning utilizing *Master Instruction.*

BOX 3.2

Teaching Excellence Curriculum Content Outline

CCN-101 Essential Guide for New Faculty Success

- Chamberlain's Community
- Chamberlain's Curricula
- Chamberlain's Learning Environment
- Chamberlain's Evaluation Processes
- Facilitators' Guide

CCN-102 Essential Guide for Clinical Faculty Success

- Curricular Foundations
- Legal and Ethical Issues
- *Master Instruction* in Clinical Education
- Student Orientation, Conferences, & Patient Care Assignments
- Clinical Evaluation Methods
- Strategies for Managing Student Misconduct and Performance Issues
- Simulation to Promote Student Learning
- Facilitators' Guide

(*continued*)

BOX 3.2

Teaching Excellence Curriculum Content Outline (*Continued*)

CCN-110 *Master Instruction:* Chamberlain Care in Action
- *Chamberlain Care* in Action
- Stories
- Reflection Journal
- *Master Instruction:* Teamwork & Reflection
- Facilitators' Guide

CCN-115 *Master Instruction:* Evidence-Based Teaching
- Learning Theories
- Transformational Teaching
- Transformational Learning
- Evidence-Based Teaching: Active, Student-Centered, Collaborative, Experimental and Problem-Based Learning
- Facilitators' Guide

CCN-120 Essential Guide for Scholarship
- Scholarship Essentials
- Scholarship at Chamberlain
- Facilitator's Guide

CCN-130 Essential Guide for Advancing Faculty Success
- Teaching With Purpose
- Grading Essentials
- Discussion Standards
- Academic Integrity
- Student Performance Issues
- Creating a *Chamberlain Care* Environment
- Facilitators' Guide

This eLearning curriculum is consistent with the National League for Nursing (NLN) Nurse Educator Competencies (NLN, 2005) and guides faculty to incorporate scholarly teaching across learning environments—clinical, classroom, and online. Like all of Chamberlain's faculty development offerings, the Teaching Excellence Curriculum incorporates *Master Instruction,* our pedagogical approach to teaching excellence. In addition, critical reflection is used to guide faculty in identifying opportunities for improvement in teaching practices, and for determining future actions and responses in the academic role (Sherwood & Horton-Deutsch, 2015). This focus on faculty learning about learning is an intentional move from traditional task-oriented training toward evidence-based professional development that places value and importance on reflection and learning-centered teaching. According to Steinert (2014), this approach to faculty development enhances transfer of learning to the professional role.

Another method to facilitate faculty learning is the use of performance-based eLearning interactives. Rahmani, Mohammadi, and Moradi (2016) report that performance-based interactives that require faculty to use information and apply skills to real-life decisions encourage learning. These performance-based activities are used throughout the Teaching Excellence Curriculum to transform static faculty development into interactive, engaging eLearning. These activities are also featured in the Teaching Excellence Concepts eRepository for just-in-time faculty development, as mentioned earlier. We use the concepts of *Master Instruction* in the development and implementation of our faculty development resources and programs as a way to model engaging teaching practices that we want faculty to exemplify.

Also included in each course in the Teaching Excellence Curriculum is a downloadable facilitators' guide to support academic leaders in leading individual and team discussions about the experiences and insights encountered while completing the course. Sherwood and Horton-Deutsch (2015) contended that reflecting together as faculty teams provides opportunity to expand perspectives, gain insights, and coordinate actions to realize change. This collective process of reflection socializes new faculty to the role, generates shared meanings, and enables different views about teaching to be shared. The questioning aspects of reflection help build a culture that nurtures ideas while cultivating individual and group awareness of expectations, values, and underlying beliefs that inform teaching practice (Sherwood & Horton-Deutsch, 2015). Hutchings, Huber, and Ciccone (2011) remarked that team reflection is foundational to transformational learning, fostering faculty inquiry and engagement. Through Chamberlain's Teaching Excellence Curriculum and a companion facilitators' guide, leaders are well supported to create a caring, collaborative community around teaching and student learning. Several leaders remarked how using the facilitators' guide provided a specific set of steps for networking and sharing of ideas to support development of new and continuing faculty. They pointed out how these guides simplified the process of how to use faculty development resources to ensure momentum in growth of the faculty team without being overwhelming. One leader reached out to offer her gratitude, saying that the Teaching Excellence Curriculum courses and facilitators' guide have bolstered her confidence and ability to guide her team in developing excellence in teaching and service. These results show in our colleague engagement scores discussed later in the chapter.

OUTCOMES OF *MASTER INSTRUCTION*

Faculty Outcomes in a Culture of Care and Service

Faculty outcome measures were constructed in alignment with our care and service values. These outcomes provide tangible goals and expectations of care behaviors relevant to the faculty role and are the basis of our performance evaluation process. Purposefully aligned with the NLN Nurse Educator Competencies (2005) and the model of scholarship of Boyer (1990), and supported by the American Association of Colleges of Nursing (2006, 2008, 2011) "essentials" documents for all degree levels, our faculty outcomes provide meaningful assessment of each faculty member's performance and inform peer observations of teaching, as well as rank and promotion criteria. In this manner, faculty outcomes guide personal and professional development, offering faculty a range of pathways to successful achievement.

Master Instruction Outcomes

As mentioned previously, early results were promising with regard to the use of *Master Instruction;* questions remained, however, whether assumptions about the benefits of *Master Instruction* would be realized with widespread adoption of this pedagogical approach. During the 2015–2016 academic year, a mixed-methods study was conducted to explore, in part, the following questions:

1. How do faculty experience *Master Instruction* and perceive its effects on teaching and learning?

2. Are there differences in observation scores among the six *Master Instruction* categories (content management, active learning, relevance, facilitation, integration, and classroom environment)?

3. What are the relationships among observation scores and selected student outcomes (mean course grade, student satisfaction with course and instructor, and student engagement index scores)?

Over the course of the academic year, 177 faculty observations were completed on 13 campuses and in the online RN-BSN completion option. Observations were conducted by peers or immediate supervisors. Observers scored faculty on how often (frequency) and how well (competency) faculty demonstrated behaviors indicative of the six *Master Instruction* categories. (See Appendix B for a description of *Master Instruction* categories and behaviors.) Scores were determined using a 1 to 5 scale, with 1 representing *never* and 5 representing *very frequently* (frequency) and 1 representing *does not meet expectations* and 5 representing *far exceeds expectations* (competency). Observers also provided an overall *Master Instruction* rating with 1 representing *very poor* and 5 representing *very good.* Descriptive and inferential statistics were used to analyze the data. Student outcomes data were collected from end-of-course surveys from the courses in which faculty observations occurred.

Qualitative data were collected from six focus groups. Four groups were comprised of campus faculty, one group from faculty teaching in the online RN-BSN track, and one group of faculty supervisors. Interviews with the groups were recorded and transcribed. Data were analyzed using hermeneutical analysis methods described by Diekelmann and Ironside (1998). Four researchers coded the data independently, then met to group codes into themes following each focus group interview. Subsequent interviews either built on existing themes or developed new themes until redundancy in themes was realized among the faculty groups. The supervisor focus group was added to illuminate the findings from the perspectives of administrators. The research team then revisited the literature on best practices for teaching and learning in higher education to inform and challenge the interpretive analysis thus far. The team concluded analysis by discerning patterns among the developed themes.

Results from the quantitative analysis showed that mean observation scores ranged from 3.38 (for competency with relevancy behaviors) to 4.27 (for frequency of content management behaviors). Online RN-BSN faculty demonstrated higher overall *Master Instruction* scores compared to campus-based BSN faculty (4.20 vs. 4.08), although this difference was not significant. Only 135 of the faculty observations were used for determination of correlations among *Master Instruction* scores and student outcomes,

TABLE 3.1

Significant Correlations Among *Master Instruction* Scores and Student Outcomes

Master Instruction Component	Student Outcome	Pearson Correlation
Content management (frequency)	Satisfaction with instructor	.196*
Content management (competency)	Course GPA	.213*
Content management (competency)	Satisfaction with course	.170*
Content management (competency)	Satisfaction with instructor	.231**
Active learning (frequency)	Satisfaction with instructor	.194*
Active learning (competency)	Satisfaction with instructor	.227**
Active learning (competency)	Student engagement	.194*
Classroom environment (frequency)	Satisfaction with instructor	.207*
Classroom environment (competency)	Satisfaction with course	.179*
Classroom environment (competency)	Satisfaction with instructor	.235**
Classroom environment (competency)	Student engagement	.206*
Overall score	Satisfaction with instructor	.204*

*$p < .05$.
**$p < .01$.

as some of the observations did not allow for anonymity of faculty performance data (e.g., only one faculty member teaching a course on any campus during a given semester). Significant findings are provided in Table 3.1.

Several important comments about these findings are warranted. Faculty varied in their ability to apply various *Master Instruction* principles in observed courses. Perhaps not surprising, faculty frequently demonstrated behaviors of effective management of course content. Such demonstration is likely influenced by the use of structured syllabi, well-planned content delivery activities, and faculty experience in the content area. Faculty were less adept with relevancy behaviors, such as using Bloom's taxonomy or other scaffolding frameworks to support deeper learning, integrate evidence and saliency into content presentation, or facilitate continuous learning. Variability in scores provides opportunities for the organization to plan future faculty development initiatives. Additional research is needed to determine if improved application of *Master Instruction* principles as noted by improved observation scores are associated with stronger influences on student outcomes.

The correlations depicted in Table 3.1 are weak, although the findings support the assertion that *Master Instruction* as an operationalization of care for students may improve student satisfaction. Further, faculty competency with active learning and classroom environment improves student engagement, and faculty competency with content management positively affects student grades. This study also found that student grade point average (GPA) was significantly correlated with student satisfaction with the course ($R = .329$, $p < .01$), student satisfaction with the instructor ($R = .263$, $p < .05$), and student engagement ($R = .216$, $p < .05$). Findings that behaviors indicative of *Master Instruction* principles positively relate to student satisfaction, engagement, and performance are congruent with those reported in the literature (e.g., Bain, 2004; Benner et al., 2010; Brookfield, 2006; DeBourgh, 2003; Mennenga, 2013; Popkess, 2010; Rowles, 2012; Russell & Slater, 2011; Smith & Roehrs, 2009). Thus, faculty behaviors related to content management, active learning, and classroom environment are important to develop and support as institutional strategies indicative of service excellence and may facilitate student success.

Of the 28 faculty members who participated in the focus groups, 16 completed a post hoc demographic survey. For these 16 faculty, the average age was 56.4 years (range 37 to 69 years). They had been RNs for an average of 31.4 years (range 14 to 48 years) and nurse educators for an average of 11.9 years (range 3 to 27 years). These 16 faculty are 87.5 percent ($n = 14$) Caucasian and 12.5 percent ($n = 2$) African American. For the most part, the participants were seasoned nurses and educators.

The participants described variable experiences and perceptions about implementing *Master Instruction* in their courses. The following patterns and descriptions were discerned from 13 themes:

> *A New Way of Thinking:* *Master Instruction* intentionally disrupts the education model at the organization. Adoption of a new way of thinking about teaching and learning, adoption of different identities as teacher and student, and new perspectives and behaviors are required. A realization occurs that learning is enhanced when faculty reflect on pedagogy and facilitative teaching behaviors, and when students place learning in a context of situation, salience, and action.

> *Making It Happen:* *Master Instruction* moves beyond theoretical understanding to application of diverse, high-impact strategies that operationalize learner-centric teaching. Learning environments suddenly look, feel, and operate differently. Environments become dynamic, adapting to learner needs and preferences as quickly as audacious creativity and teaching prowess allow. Common among these environments is heightened engagement from both student and faculty that fosters curiosity, problem solving, collaboration, and excitement with learning.

> *Challenges Abound:* Both students and faculty face substantive barriers in transforming themselves and the teaching-learning environment. Tradition, pessimism, fear, and arrogance pose barriers to change. Indeed, *Master*

Instruction is poorly suited to those too eager to acquiesce to problematic but familiar behaviors. Overcoming the challenges requires individual and organizational grit, reflection, and an abundance of support.

> **Rewards Are Plentiful:** Students and faculty quickly realize the many benefits of *Master Instruction.* Students become more engaged, ask deeper questions, perform better, and demonstrate self-accountability for learning. Faculty are more reflective, creative, and adept with in-the-moment adjustment of teaching behaviors. Faculty report a liberating joy, and new faculty readily self-identify as educators. The organization cultivates and sustains a culture of faculty excellence and positions itself as an academic reformer.

These patterns reflect a process in which both faculty and students must think differently about teaching and learning. They must cast aside traditional perspectives on the roles and accountabilities of institution, faculty, and students to forge dynamic and collaborative teams for student learning and success. Full implementation of *Master Instruction* is transformational but can only occur within an organizational culture supportive of such change. Clearly, transformation at Chamberlain is ongoing.

Participants observed the interrelated nature of *Master Instruction* and *Chamberlain Care.* Participants saw personal adoption of *Master Instruction* as a means of professional development, life-long learning, and *care for self.* They saw mentoring others, sharing *Master Instruction* resources and insights, and the institution's support for faculty development as *care for colleagues.* Additionally, participants described at length the changes they observed in the classroom. Interactions with students became livelier, students were more engaged, and performed better. Improved performance was not always shown through improved grades according to faculty, but students asked deeper questions and participated more readily in learning activities. Faculty also reported improved satisfaction ratings and student comments on end-of-course surveys. These observations support the quantitative findings of improved student satisfaction and engagement. Most importantly, faculty noted these changes as validation of *Master Instruction* as *care for students.*

The study provided us improvement opportunities. The faculty observation tool has been revised for clarity and adaptability to the online learning environment. Further research is needed to more deeply investigate how specific *Master Instruction* behaviors might influence student performance, particularly in light of the paucity of research outcomes on perceived best practices for nurse educators. Research is also needed to explore how the perceived care for self and care for colleagues aspects of *Master Instruction* affect faculty satisfaction, retention, and development.

Findings from the qualitative arm of this study have informed the faculty development team to expand *Master Instruction* offerings into a comprehensive "excellence in teaching" faculty development curriculum. Specifically, the research team noted that some faculty view *Master Instruction* simply as a set of strategies—a teaching toolkit—devoid of pedagogical underpinnings. New offerings now provide faculty a more rigorous theoretical foundation, along with greater diversity and salience in application exemplars. Early outcomes following the implementation of the Teaching Excellence Curriculum follows.

Teaching Excellence Curriculum Outcomes

To drive quality improvement, the Teaching Excellence Curriculum and other faculty development course offerings are evaluated through a strategic evaluation plan that uses the four-level model of Kirkpatrick (1994) to measure outcomes. Kirkpatrick's model is widely used across the field of health professions education, including nursing, to determine the effectiveness of professional development programs (Leslie, Baker, Egan-Lee, Esdaile, & Reeves, 2013; Opperman, Liebig, Bowling, Johnson, & Harper, 2016; Zheng, Bender, & Nadershahi, 2015). This hierarchy model evaluates outcomes of professional development, including learner satisfaction, knowledge and skill acquisition, application of new knowledge and skills, and the achievement of mission-critical goals. The four levels of evaluation determine the effectiveness of the professional development offerings in transforming learning into behavior change in participants and contributing to Chamberlain's intent to improve service and academic outcomes.

Data were captured from pre- and postcourse surveys from courses within the Teaching Excellence Curriculum across two levels: reaction and learning. A five-item Likert scale was used, with responses ranging from 1 (*strongly disagree*) to 5 (*strongly agree*). Self-reported low- and high-level outcomes were analyzed to evaluate the effectiveness of the Teaching Excellence Curriculum in preparing new faculty for the academic role. Table 3.2 reports numbers of faculty participants by program type at the time of data analysis.

Faculty participants reported a high-level of satisfaction with the professional development program (reaction; level 1 outcomes) and increased commitment to apply what was learned (learning; level 2 outcomes). The mean overall participant satisfaction and commitment scores are presented in Table 3.3. Further analysis across all four levels of evaluation will be completed as data are available, including knowledge and skill acquisition, application of new knowledge and skills, and the achievement of mission-critical goals.

TABLE 3.2

Total Participant Numbers per Course by Program Type

| Program Type | Total Participant Numbers per Course | | | | | |
	CCN-101	CCN-102	CCN-110	CCN-115	CCN-120	CCN-130
Prelicensure	308	227	185	268	221	182
RN-BSN	5	2	44	203	180	15
MSN	3	2	29	16	22	4
MSN-FNP	15	5	15	10	12	5
DNP	4	2	11	7	9	4
Total Participants	335	238	284	504	444	210

TABLE 3.3

Descriptive Statistics for Postcourse Survey Items Aligned With Kirkpatrick's Levels 1 (Satisfaction) and 2 (Commitment) of Evaluation

Kirkpatrick Level of Evaluation	Course	M	SD	N
Level 1: Reaction/Satisfaction	CCN-101	4.54	0.55	335
	CCN-102	4.65	0.54	238
	CCN-110	4.48	0.68	284
	CCN-115	4.52	0.71	504
	CCN-120	4.35	0.75	444
	CCN-130	4.57	0.58	210
Level 2: Learning/Commitment	CCN-101	4.81	0.40	335
	CCN-102	4.80	0.48	238
	CCN-110	4.79	0.44	284
	CCN-115	4.76	0.47	504
	CCN-120	4.53	0.63	444
	CCN-130	4.74	0.55	210

M, mean; SD, standard deviation; N, sample size.

Early high-level data analysis revealed an enthusiastic and substantial reach of the Teaching Excellence Curriculum across our nursing program, both prelicensure and postlicensure. Anecdotal feedback by faculty participants, solicited through campus visits and retrieved from course survey comments, was also strongly positive.

Comments from faculty participants included:

▸ This is exactly what I needed to be successful in my new role! This was a valuable curriculum and a great introduction to Chamberlain. I am excited and empowered to start as a nurse educator!

▸ I learned quite a bit of new information and clarified concepts and terms that I heard about but never really understood, especially how the concept fit into to overall plan for student success. Now that I have had this orientation, I will be proactive in taking advantage of the many rich resources that Chamberlain offers and use them to make a difference for students!

▸ This review of course content has been a formidable means to assist me to better understand my role and its application to the success of our students at Chamberlain. In doing so, I feel I am on sound footing as it relates to the integration of my teaching strategies in the classroom as well as clinical settings to achieve the overall goals of Chamberlain Care.

▸ I find Chamberlain's support and commitment to excellence motivating and empowering. I love the idea that I am working for an institution that wants not only the best from its instructors, but it wants the best for its instructors. Thank you!

> ➤ This knowledge gained will assist me as a nurse educator in performing at my best capacity and will directly impact my students.

> ➤ As a new faculty member, this was a great review of some content I knew already but now has more meaning and application. Additionally, I was not aware of some of the resources available to me that I will definitely utilize with my students.

> ➤ I have been a Chamberlain educator for almost 2 months. I'm getting ready to teach my first course in a few days and found comfort knowing that there are so many resources out there to help me!!

> ➤ Wow! This was the best preparation for a beginning educator! Thank you!

> ➤ This was a rewarding, rigorous exploration of the essentials for advancing faculty success. A "must take" for all Chamberlain Faculty!

Along with positive feedback, faculty identified time commitment as a potential barrier to completing an entire faculty development course, which typically ranges from 2 to 5 hours. Kirkpatrick and Kirkpatrick (2016) acknowledged that until barriers and challenges are addressed, development initiatives yield little impact. Lancaster, Stein, MacLean, Van Amburgh, and Persky (2014) pointed out that addressing perceived barriers demonstrates the valuing of colleague input and supports the use of resources. To this end, the Teaching Excellence Concepts, described earlier, were developed to provide a flexible mechanism to meet just-in-time requests for faculty development.

BEYOND *MASTER INSTRUCTION*: ADDITIONAL MEANS OF FACULTY SUPPORT

Beyond provision of innovative faculty development resources and training, many other initiatives have been introduced to enhance care of faculty. In May 2014, a celebratory Faculty Summit brought together faculty and interprofessional colleagues from across programs and campuses to spotlight *Master Instruction* and original faculty research. Sixteen podium and 24 poster presentations provided ample opportunities for professional development and community building, as faculty learned from and engaged in the successes of each other. In addition to exploring the latest research, discussing challenges that the profession faces, and highlighting best approaches to address those challenges, Summit attendees celebrated faculty who were recognized for their inspirational influence on students and colleagues. This meeting served as the inauguration for awarding faculty excellence, sparking abounding enthusiasm that culminated in dissemination of 11 Chamberlain awards recognizing teaching excellence, and a record-setting 414 DAISY Faculty Award nominations, most of which were student generated. An acronym for Diseases Attacking the Immune System, the DAISY Foundation™ created the DAISY Faculty Award to celebrate faculty for their impact on nursing students, patient care, and the profession of nursing.

Another means of support for faculty occurs during National Nurses Week. Faculty and nurses are honored with small gifts and a special presentation showcasing a national speaker. For example, in 2016, Susan B. Hassmiller, the director of the Future of Nursing: Campaign for Action and senior advisor for nursing with the Robert Wood Johnson Foundation, presented *A Culture of Health and the Future of Nursing,* exploring how nurses can help build a culture of health, in which good health and well-being spans across geographic, demographic, and social lines (Hassmiller, 2016).

Chamberlain faculty are also supported to explore external professional development opportunities through annual development stipends. Any faculty serving on a national organization committee or board and any faculty doing a podium presentation at a conference are fully supported in their participation, provided the organization is relevant to Chamberlain's mission and purpose. Tuition reimbursement is provided for faculty desiring to advance their education; tuition is free for all Chamberlain programs, and up to $50,000 is reimbursed for doctoral education.

In addition to national initiatives to support faculty, each campus/program leader honors faculty accomplishment in different ways. For example, postlicensure leaders acknowledge outstanding faculty achievement in *Care Connection,* a newsletter for our online faculty. Leaders also recognize faculty feats, including presentations and publications, in our weekly college newsletter, *Chamberlain Pulse.*

FACULTY ENGAGEMENT AND CARING CLIMATE

To ensure that our cultural transformation is positively supporting faculty, outcomes related to faculty care are regularly gathered. Chamberlain surveys all colleagues annually on their perspectives of Chamberlain as an employer, how well the organization meets their needs, and their relationships with supervisors and other colleagues. The Colleague Engagement Survey administered by Spring International (2017) was administered until fall 2016 to encourage frank employee input and allow findings to be benchmarked against large external samples. The survey provides an overall engagement score, based on a 100-point scale, that summarizes colleagues' overall perspectives of a caring and supportive workplace climate. An abridged version of the survey was typically administered midway through the year as a means to track findings more regularly and to assess the impact of initiatives directed at improving engagement.

Table 3.4 depicts overall engagement scores from faculty over the past few years. Scores peaked in 2012 and 2014 when faculty were brought to national Summit meetings on *Chamberlain Care* and other professional development topics. Scores dipped in fall 2012 with the implementation of a new curriculum and again in fall 2015 when the college made a significant change in its NCLEX success program that was followed by challenges with first-time pass rates on the nursing licensure examination. Since 2013, scores have remained above benchmark for the best U.S. companies and continue to rival benchmark scores for the best companies in the world.

The vendor for the Colleague Engagement Survey was changed in fall 2016 to Korn Ferry Hay Group, which uses a different survey methodology where employee engagement is only one measure of overall employee effectiveness. A survey using the new vendor was conducted in fall 2016; Chamberlain results are still at or above both the high performing and global norms.

Although the Colleague Engagement Survey includes a caring index score derived from several survey items, the proprietary survey does not accommodate deeper exploration of faculty perspectives on possible outcomes of *Chamberlain Care.* In 2015, Chamberlain was afforded the opportunity to use the Caring Characteristics Within School of Nursing Climate (C_2SNC) survey, a new tool with established content validity and high internal consistency reliability (McDaniel, Schlosser, & Hayne, 2014). This 28-item survey measures characteristics of a caring nursing academic environment on

TABLE 3.4

Overall Faculty Engagement Scores Compared to National and Global Benchmarks

Date	Chamberlain University College of Nursing	U.S. Best Companies	Global Best Companies
May 2011	63	65	72
Sept. 2011	73	65	72
May 2012	75	65	72
Sept. 2012	61	65	72
May 2013	70	65	72
May 2014	73	65	72
Oct. 2014	72	65	72
May 2015	70	65	72
Nov. 2015	67	65	72
May 2016	72	66	72

a seven-point scale, with higher scores reflecting stronger levels of agreement that a caring characteristic is present. Scores are tabulated for each item and for each of four dimensions: teamwork/trust, support, feeling valued, and respect. In April 2015, Chamberlain sent the survey to all colleagues, receiving 854 surveys for analysis (response rate of 41.5 percent). Faculty provided 426 of the surveys (full time = 217; part time = 209) for analysis; mean dimension scores were calculated from surveys in which all dimension survey items were completed. Of the faculty responders, 93.2 percent were female; 77.3 percent were Caucasian; 48.3 percent were doctorally prepared; and 82.7 percent had been employed for less than 5 years at Chamberlain, but 59.6 percent had taught for more than 5 years prior to employment at Chamberlain. Part-time faculty rated Chamberlain more highly in caring characteristics for each of the four dimensions. The differences were significant at the level of $p < .001$ for *feeling valued* and *respect*. (See Table 3.5.)

One explanation for the higher ratings by part-time faculty is that they do not carry the nonteaching responsibilities of full-time faculty. It is noteworthy, however, that the literature suggests that part-time faculty often report general dissatisfaction and feeling devalued (Dolan, 2011; Forbes, Hickey, & White, 2010). The findings from this analysis suggest that a culture of care at Chamberlain is evident to part-time faculty, many of whom are employed as nurses or faculty elsewhere.

Mean dimension scores were then compared to a national faculty sample provided by the tool's developers at Samford University. As noted in Table 3.6, Chamberlain faculty rated the workplace environment significantly higher than the national sample in all caring climate dimensions.

TABLE 3.5

Mean Total Dimension Scores on the C₂SNC Survey: Comparison Between Chamberlain Full-Time and Part-Time Faculty

Dimension	Full-Time Faculty	Part-Time Faculty
Trust/Teamwork	80.99 (SD = 15.55)	82.17* (SD = 15.62)
Score range = 14 to 98	n = 174	n = 201
Support	44.28 (SD = 5.09)	45.19* (SD = 5.50)
Score range = 7 to 49	n = 175	n = 204
Feeling valued	22.10 (SD = 6.15)	24.37** (SD = 4.69)
Score range = 4 to 28	n = 175	n = 204
Respect	18.44 (SD = 2.86)	19.64** (SD = 2.52)
Score range = 3 to 21	n = 177	n = 216

SD, standard deviation; n, sample size.
*Not significant.
**p < .001.

'Additional data analysis determined which survey items most predicted Chamberlain faculty scores. Seven items were identified that account for 70 percent of the variance related to perceptions of a caring climate. These items are noted in Table 3.7 in rank order of relative weight. It is noteworthy that these survey items are consistent with care for colleagues and care for students in the *Chamberlain Care* Model.

TABLE 3.6

Mean Total Dimension Scores on the C₂SNC Survey: Comparison Between Chamberlain and National Faculty Samples

Dimension	Chamberlain University College of Nursing Faculty	National Faculty Sample
Trust/Teamwork	81.18* (SD = 15.91)	77.14 (SD = 15.88)
Score range = 14 to 98	n = 387	n = 1,955
Support	44.68* (SD = 5.40)	43.24 (SD = 5.37)
Score range = 7 to 49	n = 391	n = 2,009
Feeling valued	23.18* (SD = 5.58)	22.07 (SD = 5.22)
Score range = 4 to 28	n = 392	n = 2,045
Respect	19.05* (SD = 2.83)	17.60 (SD = 3.31)
Score range = 3 to 21	n = 414	n = 2,097

SD, standard deviation, n, sample size.
*p < .001.

TABLE 3.7

Caring Characteristics Predicting Chamberlain Faculty's Perceptions of a Caring Climate: Items From the C_2SNC Survey

Survey Item	Beta
Faculty feel their contributions are valued	0.323*
Faculty feel supported to grow	0.269***
Faculty are concerned for students	0.222*
Director/Dean is concerned about faculty	0.134***
Student opinions are valued	0.122**
Director/Dean is concerned about students	0.121**
Faculty are consistent in their interactions	0.086***

*$p < .001$.
**$p < .01$.
***$p < .05$.

Prior to administration of the C_2SNC survey, Chamberlain had become interested in the work of the DAISY Foundation and its expanded recognition of nurse educators and excellence in teaching. Congruent with *Chamberlain Care* and Chamberlain's emphasis on care for colleagues, the DAISY Foundation provides explicit recognition of faculty accomplishments through publication in newsletters, blogs, and local press, through announcements at meetings, and through awards programs. Chamberlain participates in both the DAISY Faculty Award program, as well as DAISY in Training recognition of students who demonstrate caring behaviors to patients and families. Both Chamberlain and the DAISY Foundation were interested in learning how faculty perceived the value and impact of recognition. To that end, Chamberlain included four items as a separate section that accompanied the C_2SNC survey:

> Recognition efforts contribute to colleagues feeling cared for by Chamberlain.

> Recognition efforts are clearly linked to *Chamberlain Care* core values.

> Recognition efforts at Chamberlain motivate faculty and colleagues to give their best effort.

> Overall, I am satisfied with recognition efforts that reward my work effort at Chamberlain.

Pearson's product-moment correlation coefficients were calculated to examine relationships between the recognition effort items with overall dimension scores on the C_2SNC survey. All items were significantly correlated with each of the four caring climate dimensions at the $p < .001$ level. The strength of correlations was moderate for the *respect, support,* and *trust/teamwork* caring dimensions ($R = .4$ to $.6$) and strong for the *value* caring dimension ($R = .7$ to $.9$) (Dancey & Reidy, 2004). It is noteworthy that these findings are congruent with the C_2SNC survey item that carries the greatest predictive value, "Faculty feel their contributions are valued." The importance of recognizing faculty accomplishments as a relatively facile method to support a caring climate cannot be understated. Plans are currently under way at Chamberlain to collaborate with the DAISY Foundation to research the meaning, perceived value, and possible outcomes of faculty recognition.

Creating a culture of care and service has brought Chamberlain many opportunities to celebrate successes as we make progress in creating the kind of environment where faculty want to work and students feel cared for as they make their passion for nursing a reality. Along with our successes, we have faced many challenges and opportunities for improvement.

CHALLENGES AND OPPORTUNITIES IN CARE FOR FACULTY

Change is seldom without challenge. Successfully transforming and sustaining a culture of care for faculty and students requires a deliberate shift in perception of challenge as an obstacle to challenge as an opportunity for innovation. When challenges are leveraged as opportunities, opportunities abound for creative solutions. Promoting teaching excellence in a culture of care called for nothing less than entrepreneurial thinking in developing a faculty development program to efficiently, effectively, and economically transform teaching practice for a large, diverse cadre of faculty across Chamberlain programs and learning environments.

An entrepreneurial mind-set requires agile thinking, resourcefulness when approaching new problems, sharing ideas freely, and viewing challenges as learning and growing experiences (Pucciarelli & Kaplan, 2016). Being entrepreneurial can mean simply thinking outside of the box and expecting the unexpected. This ability to work around issues and find new ways was essential in developing the Teaching Excellence Curriculum, which is a relatively new offering at Chamberlain.

Prior to these resources, our prelicensure campuses approached new hire orientation through varied processes and with a range of results, whereas our postlicensure programs had effective program-specific orientations. None, however, placed emphasis on the development of teaching competencies beyond basic skills. Ensuring success and satisfaction in the academic role is essential to prepare new educators and assist them in their professional development (Felver et al., 2010). Although our goal to transition new faculty across the first year of teaching was clear, the process steps were not. New educators bring varying education and teaching experience to their new role, and different levels of students and learning environments require specific skill sets. A standardized curriculum fell short of fulfilling the diverse learning needs of our faculty.

To meet this challenge, the first two courses of the Teaching Excellence Curriculum were developed to provide competencies foundational to the academic role: the Essential Guide for New Faculty Success and the Essential Guide for New Clinical Faculty Success. These courses were used to orient new faculty on Chamberlain campuses, whereas our online programs integrated essential content into their preexisting, program-specific orientations. Through this approach, the new faculty success courses provided a customizable pathway for learning. Each course incorporated extractable eLearning interactives to promote varied opportunities for enhanced learning experiences to meet individual and program needs. Academic leaders determine the use, structure, and sequence of these interactives, taking into account the experience, knowledge, and learning goals of the faculty member, making personalized learning a reality. Additionally, these eLearning interactives can be used to facilitate live or virtual, individual and/or collective discussions to enhance learning or address deficiencies. These new courses were also designed to be easily adapted for live implementation on our campuses with step-by-step suggestions for facilitation provided in the companion facilitators' guide.

Development of these two courses required flexibility and working toward a goal yet being able to adapt to changing circumstances. We learned to see opportunities in not-so-obvious places, as we implemented solutions to address the applicability of these virtual resources to meet a range of faculty learning needs and locations. Following the successful launch of these courses, and informed by course evaluation data, the remaining courses in Teaching Excellence Curriculum were developed using similar design methods to advance the scholarship of teaching. With the design process in place, new challenges were then faced regarding competencies needed to ensure continuing success in the academic role.

Successful teaching requires skills beyond an advanced education and clinical expertise to prepare future nurses for their roles in an ever-changing and complex health care arena. However, there exists a dearth of nursing literature regarding developing educator competencies to support and guide continued growth and development in the educator role. Although the NLN's Core Competencies for Nurse Educators (2005) gave voice to the requisite knowledge necessary to provide excellent nursing education, this definitive set of standards does not address continuous quality improvement in the nurse educator role (Halstead, 2007). Furthermore, little is known about what methods effectively socialize nurses into the role of educator or facilitate ongoing role development along the career trajectory (Fairbrother, Rafferty, Woods, Tyler, & Howell, 2015; Kuiper, 2012). Our commitment to advancing scholarly teaching required developing, using, and testing *Master Instruction* instructional methods for incorporation in the Teaching Excellence Curriculum. Developing and evaluating a comprehensive faculty development plan is essential in creating a culture of teaching excellence that is grounded in theory and data.

Opportunities to think in new ways did not end with the development of Teaching Excellence Curriculum. Implementation of these resources also required an entrepreneurial mind-set. Developing the teaching capacity of the individual faculty member in a supportive culture entailed further experimenting with solutions and measuring outcomes. Faculty development is contextual and succeeds only when it is designed to value teaching, reawaken motivation and enthusiasm, and improve knowledge, skills, and abilities (Lancaster et al., 2014). Implementation of faculty development initiatives posed a considerable challenge for a small national team of people who live in different states and who service pre-and postlicensure programs that employ more than 2,000 full- and part-time faculty across learning environments. To meet this challenge, the faculty development team equipped academic leaders to effectively use the Teaching Excellence Comprehensive Program to contextualize learning and support faculty teaching and development at their location or program. Regional immersions were held to engage leaders in knowledge and resource sharing, enhancing their capacity to serve as stewards of teaching excellence.

Alertness to opportunity led to other creative solutions to support faculty in their professional growth. Recognizing and valuing faculty time commitments at work and at home, as well as the unique learning environments in which they work, the courses in Teaching Excellence Curriculum provide continuing education through an external accredited provider. Courses are developed providing logical in-course breaks to facilitate completion in one or multiple sittings. By allowing for a self-paced format, faculty are able to progress through a course based on their perceived competency in a given area. Additional resources are provided for varied learner preferences, including text and audio options, provision of course transcripts, and the inclusion of significant resources to expand learning, allowing faculty to download aspects of the eLearning interactive in static format for future reference. Most courses contain multiple exemplars to contextualize learning across environments. Faculty select the learning environment—clinical, classroom, or online—to facilitate application of the content through direct participation in scenarios relevant to everyday teaching.

Most, if not all, of the resources mentioned previously were identified and requested by faculty to add value to their professional growth. Designing and implementing the requested resources propelled innovation, stretching our capacity to bring their ideas to reality. Close collaboration with faculty and seizing opportunities and discovering and creating solutions were fundamental to enriching the life and work of faculty and promoting teaching excellence in a culture of care.

THE FUTURE

A reflective look back reveals our accomplishment in creating a care culture through faculty preparation, support, and development. Developed faculty consider the student, the environment, the course, and the materials used in the teaching interaction. Although we have addressed the student, environment, and faculty, we see opportunity to further enhance our courses and course materials as we complete our intentional shift from a faculty-focused to a student-focused approach. This shift has emerged as a holistic approach to designing a learning-centered curriculum, which serves as a framework for a *Chamberlain Care* curriculum. This holistic model pivots from teaching to learning with a focus on student engagement, and includes support resources, adaptive content, and dynamic connections with peers and faculty.

The current state of our curriculum places dependency on faculty to choose appropriate learning strategies for the course and learner. In addition, students are required to self-identify needs and seek out support. Student learning support, success preparation, and resources reside in multiple areas within the college and the program. With increased awareness of the needs of our diverse students and a complex fast-paced program, there is little time to misstep. The proposed course framework will be adaptable and flexible to fit individual student needs while supporting program outcomes.

The culture of *Chamberlain Care* continues to drive change in the interactions between faculty and student. Our future is to create a *Chamberlain Care* curriculum that empowers students as equal participants, supported by prepared faculty, that is aligned with our culture.

References

American Association of Colleges of Nursing. (2006). *The essentials of doctoral education for advanced nursing practice.* Washington, DC: Author. Retrieved June 19, 2017, from http://www.aacn.nche.edu/dnp/Essentials.pdf

American Association of Colleges of Nursing. (2008). *The essentials of baccalaureate education for professional nursing practice.* Washington, DC: Author. Retrieved June 19, 2017, from http://www.aacn.nche.edu/education-resources/BaccEssentials08.pdf

American Association of Colleges of Nursing. (2011). *The essentials of master's education in nursing.* Washington, DC: Author. Retrieved June 19, 2017, from http://www.aacn.nche.edu/education-resources/MastersEssentials11.pdf

Ardisson, M., Smallheer, B., Moore, G., & Christenbery, T. (2015). Meta-evaluation: Experiences in an accelerated graduate nurse education program. *Journal of Professional Nursing, 31*(6), 508–515. Available at http://www.professionalnursing.org/article/S8755-7223(15)00054-X/fulltext

Atkinson, D. J., & Bolt, S. (2010). Using teaching observations to reflect upon and improve teaching practice in higher education. *Journal of the Scholarship of Teaching and Learning, 10*(3), 1–19.

Bain, K. (2004). *What the best college teachers do.* Cambridge, MA: Harvard University Press.

Banks, P., Waugh, A., Henderson, J., Sharp, B., Brown, M., Oliver, J., et al. (2014). Enriching the care of patients with dementia in acute settings? The Dementia Champions Programme in Scotland. *Dementia, 13*(6), 717–736. doi:10.1177/1471301213485084

Bass, R. (2012). Disrupting ourselves: The problem of learning in higher education. *EDUCAUSE Review.* Retrieved June 19, 2017, from https://er.educause.edu/articles/2012/3/disrupting-ourselves-the-problem-of-learning-in-higher-education

Benner, P., Sutphen, M., Leonard, V., & Day, L. (2010). *Educating nurses: A call for radical transformation.* San Francisco: Jossey-Bass.

Boyer, E. L. (1990). *Scholarship reconsidered: Priorities of the professoriate.* Lawrenceville, NJ: Princeton University Press.

Brett, A. L., Branstetter, J. E., & Wagner, P. D. (2014). Nurse educators' perceptions of caring attributes in current and ideal work environments. *Nursing Education Perspectives, 35*(6), 360–366. doi:10.5480/13-1113.1

Brookfield, S. D. (2006). *The skillful teacher: On technique, trust, and responsiveness in the classroom* (2nd ed.). San Francisco: Wiley & Sons.

Candela, L., Gutierrez, A. P., & Keating, S. (2015). What predicts nurse faculty members' intent to stay in the academic organization? A structural equation model of a national survey of nursing faculty. *Nurse Education Today, 35*(4), 580–589. Available at http://www.nurseeducationtoday.com/article/S0260-6917(15)00002-7/fulltext

Dancey, C. P., & Reidy, J. (2004). *Statistics without maths for psychology* (3rd ed.). Upper Saddle River, NJ: Prentice Hall.

DeBourgh, G. A. (2003). Predictors of student satisfaction in distance-delivered graduate nursing courses: What matters most? *Journal of Professional Nursing, 19*(3), 149–162. Available at http://www.professionalnursing.org/article/S8755-7223(03)00072-3/fulltext

Diekelmann, N., & Ironside, P. M. (1998). Preserving writing in doctoral education: Exploring the concernful practices of schooling learning teaching. *Journal of Advanced Nursing, 28*(6), 1347–1355.

Dolan, V. (2011). The isolation of online adjunct faculty and its impact on their performance. *International Review of Research in Open and Distance Learning, 12*(2), 62–77. Available at http://www.irrodl.org/index.php/irrodl/article/view/793

Fairbrother, G., Rafferty, R., Woods, A., Tyler, V., & Howell, W. (2015). Commencing a nurse education role development journey in a regional Australian health district: Results from a mixed method baseline inquiry. *Journal of Nursing and Education and*

Practice, 5(8), 7–16. Available at http://www.sciedupress.com/journal/index.php/jnep/article/view/6624

Felver, F., Gaines, B., Heims, M., Lasater, K., Lausten, G., Lynch, M., et al. (2010). *Best practices in teaching and learning in nursing education.* New York: National League for Nursing.

Forbes, M. O., Hickey, M. T., & White, J. (2010). Adjunct faculty development: Reported needs and innovative solutions. *Journal of Professional Nursing, 20*(2), 116–124. Available at http://www.professionalnursing.org/article/S8755-7223(09)00120-3/fulltext

Forneris, S. G., & Fey, M. K. (2016). Critical conversations: The NLN guide for teaching thinking. *Nursing Education Perspectives, 37*(5), 248–249. doi:10.1097/01.NEP.0000000000000069

Grealish, L., Henderson, A., Quero, F., Phillips, R., & Surawski, M. (2015). The significance of 'facilitator as a change agent'–organizational learning culture in aged care home settings. *Journal of Clinical Nursing, 24*(7-8), 961–969. doi:10.1111/jocn.12656

Halstead, J. (2007). *Nurse educator competencies: Creating an evidence-based practice for nurse educators.* New York: National League for Nursing.

Hassmiller, S. (2016). *Susan Hassmiller Presentation on Advancing a Culture of Health.* Chamberlain College of Nursing and Robert Wood Johnson Foundation. Retrieved June 19, 2017, from https://www.youtube.com/watch?v=aCficTtRZ1I&feature=youtu.be

Hutchings, P., Huber, M. T., & Ciccone, A. (2011). *The scholarship of teaching and learning reconsidered: Institutional integration and impact.* San Francisco: Jossey-Bass.

Jasimuddin, S. M., & Hasan, I. (2015). Organizational culture, structure, technology infrastructure and knowledge sharing: Empirical evidence from MNCs based in Malaysia. *Vine, 45*(1), 67–88. Available at http://www.emeraldinsight.com/doi/abs/10.1108/VINE-05-2014-0037

Jornsay, D. L., & Garnett, E. D. (2014). Diabetes champions: Culture change through education. *Diabetes Spectrum, 27*(3), 188–192. doi:10.2337/diaspect.27.3.188

Kaasalainen, S., Ploeg, J., Donald, F., Coker, E., Brazil, K., Martin-Misener, R., et al. (2015). Positioning clinical nurse specialists and nurse practitioners as change champions to implement a pain protocol in long-term care. *Pain Management Nursing, 16*(2), 78–88. Available at http://www.painmanagementnursing.org/article/S1524-9042(14)00049-6/fulltext

Kirkpatrick, D. L. (1994). *Evaluating training programs: The four levels.* San Francisco: Berrett-Koehler Publishers.

Kirkpatrick, J. D., & Kirkpatrick, W. K. (2016). *Kirkpatrick's four levels of training evaluation.* Alexandria, VA: Association for Talent Development.

Kopelman, M., & Vayndorf, M. (2012). Self-reflection on undergraduate teaching. *Academic Exchange Quarterly, 16*(4), 17.

Kuiper, R. (2012). Expanding the repertoire of teaching and learning strategies for nurse educators: Introducing interpretive pedagogies in an online graduate nurse education course. *Nursing Education Perspectives, 33*(5), 342–345.

Lancaster, J. W., Stein, S. M., MacLean, L. G., Van Amburgh, J., & Persky, A. M. (2014). Faculty development program models to advance teaching and learning within health science programs. *American Journal of Pharmaceutical Education, 78*(5), 99. doi:10.5688/ajpe78599

Leslie, K., Baker, L., Egan-Lee, E., Esdaile, M., & Reeves, S. (2013). Advancing faculty development in medical education: A systematic review. *Academic Medicine, 88*(7), 1038–1045. doi:10.1097/ACM.0b013e318294fd29

McDaniel, G. S., Schlosser, S. P., & Hayne, A. N. (2014, September). *The Caring Characteristics within School of Nursing (C2SNC) Instrument.* Poster presented at the National League for Nursing Summit, Phoenix, AZ.

Mennenga, H. A. (2013). Student engagement and examination performance in a team-based learning course. *Journal of Nursing Education, 52*(8), 475–479. doi:10.3928/01484834-20130718-04

Merillat, L., & Scheibmeir, M. (2016). Developing a quality improvement process to optimize faculty success. *Online Learning*. Retrieved June 19, 2017, from https://olj.onlinelearningconsortium.org/index.php/olj/article/view/977

Mount, A., & Anderson, I. (2015). Driving change—Not just a walk in the park: The role of the nurse champion in sustained change. *Nurse Leader, 13*(4), 36–38. Available at http://www.nurseleader.com/article/S1541-4612(15)00166-4/fulltext

National League for Nursing Task Group on Nurse Educator Competencies. (2005). *Competencies for nurse educators.* New York: Author.

National Research Council Committee on Developments in the Science of Learning. (2000). *How people learn: Brain, mind, experience, and school: Expanded edition.* Washington, DC: National Academies Press.

Opperman, C., Liebig, D., Bowling, J., Johnson, C. S., & Harper, M. (2016). Measuring return on investment for professional development activities: Implications for practice. *Journal for Nurses in Professional Development, 32*(4), 176–184. doi:10.1097/NND.0000000000000274

Paradeise, C., & Thoenig, J. C. (2013). Academic institutions in search of quality: Local orders and global standards. *Organization Studies, 34*(2), 189–218.

Peters, M. A., & Boylston, M. (2006). Mentoring adjunct faculty: Innovative solutions. *Nurse Educator, 31*(2), 61–64.

Popkess, A. M. (2010). *The relationship between undergraduate, baccalaureate nursing student engagement and use of active learning strategies in the classroom.* (Doctoral dissertation). Retrieved from ProQuest Dissertations and Theses. (Accession No. 3397470.)

Pucciarelli, F., & Kaplan, A. (2016). Competition and strategy in higher education: Managing complexity and uncertainty. *Business Horizons, 59*(3), 311–320. Available at http://www.sciencedirect.com/science/article/pii/S0007681316000045?via%3Dihub

Rahmani, A., Mohammadi, A., & Moradi, Y. (2016). Effectiveness of scenario-based education on the performance of the nurses in the critical cardiac care unit for patients with acute coronary syndrome. *Health Sciences, 5*(8), 218–224.

Roberts, K. K., Chrisman, S. K., & Flowers, C. (2013). The perceived needs of nurse clinicians as they move into an adjunct clinical faculty role. *Journal of Professional Nursing, 29*(5), 295–301. Available at http://www.professionalnursing.org/article/S8755-7223(12)00198-6/fulltext

Rogers, E. M. (2010). *Diffusion of innovations* (4th ed.). New York: Simon & Schuster.

Rowles, C. J. (2012). Strategies to promote critical thinking and active learning. In D. M. Billings & J. A. Halstead (Eds.), *Teaching in nursing: A guide for faculty* (4th ed.; pp. 258–284). St. Louis, MO: Elsevier.

Russell, B., & Slater, G. R. L. (2011). Factors that encourage student engagement: Insights from a case study of 'first-time' students in a New Zealand university. *Journal of University Teaching and Learning Practice, 8*(1), article 7. Available at http://ro.uow.edu.au/jutlp/vol8/iss1/7

Sabelli, N., & Dede, C. (2013). Empowering design-based implementation research: The need for infrastructure. In B. J. Fishman, W. R. Penuel, A.-R. Allen, & B. H. Cheng (Eds.), *Design-based implementation research: Theories, methods, and exemplars* (pp. 464–480). Yearbook of the National Society for the Study of Education. New York: Teachers College, Columbia University.

Sarikaya, O., Kalaca, S., Yegen B. C., & Cali, S. (2010). The impact of a faculty development program: Evaluation based on the self-assessment of medical educators from preclinical and clinical disciplines. *Advances in Physiology Education, 34*(2), 35–40. doi:10.1152/advan.00024.2010

Schaefer, K. M., & Zygmont, D. (2003). Analyzing the teaching style of nursing faculty: Does it promote a student-centered or teacher-centered learning environment? *Nursing Education Perspectives, 24*(5), 238–245.

Schoening, A. M. (2013). From bedside to classroom: The nurse educator transition model. *Nursing Education Perspectives, 34*(3), 167–172.

Sherwood, G., & Horton-Deutsch, S. (2015). *Reflective organizations: On the front lines of QSEN and reflective practice implementation.* Indianapolis, IN: Sigma Theta Tau Press.

Smith, S. J., & Roehrs, C. J. (2009). High fidelity simulation: Factors correlated with nursing student satisfaction and self-confidence. *Nursing Education Perspectives, 30*(2), 74–78.

Spring International. (2017). Home page: *Surveys*. Retrieved June 19, 2017, from http://www.springitl.com

Steinert, Y. (Ed.). (2014). Faculty development: Future directions. In *Faculty development in the health professions* (pp. 421–442). Dordrecht, Netherlands: Springer.

Steinert, Y., Mann, K., Anderson, B., Barnett, B. M., Centeno, A., Naismith, L., et al. (2016). A systematic review of faculty development initiatives designed to enhance teaching effectiveness: A 10-year update: BEME Guide No. 40. *Medical Teacher, 38*(8), 769–786. Available at http://www.tandfonline.com/doi/full/10.1080/0142159X.2016.1181851

Vyas, R., Faith, M., Selvakumar, D., Pulimood, A., & Lee, M. (2016). Project-based faculty development for e-learning. *Clinical Teacher, 13*(6), 405–410. doi:10.1111/tct.12486

Witte, T. C. H., & Jansen, E. P. W. A. (2016). Students' voice on literature teacher excellence: Towards a teacher-organized model of continuing professional development. *Teaching and Teacher Education, 56*, 162–172. Available at http://www.sciencedirect.com/science/article/pii/S0742051x16300361?via%3Dihub

Zheng, M., Bender, D., & Nadershahi, N. (2015). Faculty professional development in emergent pedagogies for instructional innovation in dental education. *European Journal of Dental Education, 21*(2), 67–78. doi:10.1111/eje.12180

4

A Culture of Care for Students

W. Richard Cowling, III, PhD, AHN-BC, FAAN, ANEF
Linda Hollinger-Smith, PhD, RN, FAAN, ANEF
Carole R. Eldridge, DNP, RN, CNE, NEA-BC

"What is more important than knowledge?" asked the Mind.
"Caring and seeing with the heart," answered the Soul.
—Flavia

As described in Chapter 1, *Chamberlain Care* evolved from an initiative focused on service excellence to an integrated, holistic educational model that incorporates the core ideals of care for self, care for colleagues, and care for students. The learning environment provides a quality academic experience and support services to help diverse students become extraordinary nurses, focusing on three essential aims (Chamberlain University College of Nursing, 2017):

> ▸ **To Educate:** A culture of care creates an academic environment in which students thrive by being appreciated for their wholeness and individuality and supported to discover and unlock their potential.

> ▸ **To Empower:** Teaching is an enterprise of engagement and collaboration between students and faculty that fosters accountability and self-determination in the practice of nursing.

> ▸ **To Embolden:** The learning environment is intentionally designed to promote and instill confidence in one's professional identity as a nurse.

The Chamberlain leadership took seriously the education of students through empowering and emboldening them to become extraordinary nurses. *Chamberlain Care* embodies student care that promotes self-determination, accountability, confidence, and courage, which we believe is essential to extraordinary nursing. As a critical element of the cultural transformation, we knew it would involve engaging in education and consciousness raising throughout the organization.

Improving student support extended across all program levels, serving the distinct needs of both prelicensure and postlicensure students. We made sure that *Chamberlain Care* accounted for differences in content delivery methods, particularly as related to the postlicensure online environment and prelicensure campus environment. Postlicensure students rarely meet each other or faculty in person, living and working in widely varying geographic regions, so building a caring community presents different challenges. Further, the students themselves bring different characteristics, views, and experiences to their education at different points in their educational careers.

CARE AND STUDENT SUCCESS

Beck (2001) conducted a metasynthesis of literature on caring among faculty, faculty–student caring, caring among nursing students, and nursing student–patient caring. She concluded that creating a caring environment impacts how students care for patients, and students and faculty experience caring as a contagious experience that provokes a strong desire to care for others.

Wade and Kasper (2006) reported that student–faculty caring relationships help students grow as caring professional nurses. Simmons and Cavanaugh (2000) conducted a quantitative study of female nursing students showing school climate to be the strongest predictor of postgraduate caring ability. The researchers advocated attention to more caring climates in nursing education.

Hoffman (2014) examined literature on student–faculty relationships and the contexts in which they occur at 4-year colleges and universities to ascertain their purported significance to persistence and completion. Although the literature suggests that there are major challenges in navigating the landscape of student–faculty relationships, including the need for clarity in boundaries, there are great benefits to attending to them. "A steadfast focus on student academic success requires [that] faculty engage in positive and supportive relationships in academic contexts, especially in the classroom" (p. 18). Hoffman also noted the importance of individualizing and contextualizing relationships to accommodate the student's strengths and needs. Hoffman does not refer to the concept of caring; however, these characteristics are associated with caring faculty–student interactions described in earlier phenomenologic studies (Cohen, 1998; Dillon & Stines, 1996).

Data on 385 nursing students enrolled in a first medical-surgical course across seven undergraduate campuses in Texas were analyzed in part to examine the influence of students' perceptions of faculty caring on academic performance (Torregosa, Ynalvez, & Morin, 2015). The results of this study demonstrated that the "student perception of faculty caring, specifically faculty having a positive outlook and compassion, enhanced student performance" (p. 865). Miller (2007) conducted a study of 203 college students to examine faculty–student relations for caring behaviors, and to determine if a student's relationship with faculty made a difference in his or her ability to persist in school. The research demonstrated that significant faculty relationships were important to student retention, and those relationships were characterized by 13 dimensions of caring based on a scale developed by the researcher.

McEnroe-Pettite (2011) built a case that faculty caring in the form of general support is beneficial for at-risk students in the areas of retention and academic success. Likewise, Bankert and Kozel (2005) advocated for caring learning environments for adult nursing students. They describe a project involving a small group of students using reflective practice and student–faculty partnerships. The characteristics of a caring learning environment that emerged from the group were valuing, genuine dialogue, relations, and connectedness. Key aspects of the learning experience were attentiveness and openness to one another and meaningful relationships and appreciation for colleagues.

From legal studies, Pattison, Hale, and Gowens (2011) make the case that caring is an essential aspect of excellent education: "Students are more likely to be satisfied and successful in classes where they perceive that professors care about them as individuals rather than merely focusing on the transfer of knowledge" (p. 39). Using a variety of strategies including literature review, the critical incident technique, student responses, and characteristics of excellent professors, Pattison and colleagues aimed to determine which teaching behaviors are most perceived as caring. They believe you teach teachers to be excellent by focusing on the behaviors that matter. The results of their exhaustive study showed myriad behaviors that students associated with a caring professor. However, the one behavior that seemed to dominate was "appreciation of professors who will let students know them as individuals" (p. 63). There were four categories of behavior described in detail that reflected excellent teaching: affirmation of students, taking time, the teaching task (method and style of teaching), and communication techniques.

There is a small body of emerging literature regarding caring in the online learning environment in contrast to the classroom. In a small study ($N = 48$) of RN-BSN completion students from historically black colleges, the researchers sought to determine the participants' preferred instructor caring behaviors in an online environment (Mann, 2014). All respondents believed that a caring environment could be created, and most believed that it had an impact on their success. The most important elements of a caring online learning environment were "(1) attention to detail in organization and clarity; (2) prompt and detailed feedback on assignments, and (3) prompt response to students' questions" (p. 33).

Sitzman (2016) conducted a study of 56 online nursing instructors from 10 states and 20 institutions aimed at describing instructors' responses to students' needs for caring. Sitzman concluded that "the combined results of this and other studies about caring in online courses provide validation from both instructor and student perspectives that genuine caring can be effectively conveyed through mindful attention, lovingkindness, compassionate awareness, courteousness, mercy, and appreciation for the humanity of self and others" (p. 70).

Plante and Asselin (2014) conducted a literature review "to identify the best practices and evidence-based strategies for creating an online learning environment that encompasses caring behaviors and promotes social presence" (p. 219). The results showed that caring behaviors and social presence in the online environment is fostered when faculty exchanges are respectful; encouraging; timely; and frequently offer caring interactions, mutual respect, and meaningful relationship building.

In summary, the literature of the phenomena of care and caring in education is sparse and built mainly on qualitative research and literature reviews. The studies that do exist rely mainly on student perceptions of what constitutes caring in education, and the characteristics gleaned from the literature are not concise and clear. This is epitomized in the study by Pattison et al. (2011). They report that "one of the most interesting results of the study was the realization that students will perceive almost everything a professor does as a reflection of the professor's level of caring and respect for students" (p. 52). There is overriding agreement that caring student–faculty relationships and caring learning environments make a positive impact on student retention, academic success, and student satisfaction. There is some support for what constitutes caring in an online environment. Yet taking the literature as a whole, there are major gaps in consistently conceptualizing and measuring caring climates and caring faculty characteristics beyond self-report or logical argumentation based on critical analysis of literature. We believe that our efforts to implement *Chamberlain Care,* monitor key student, graduate, and faculty outcome metrics, and conduct research have the potential to advance the body of knowledge of the meaningfulness and efficacy of a caring learning culture and caring teaching.

From Susan King, Chicago campus president:

> As I exited Stroger Hospital after visiting Phil (a student who was hospitalized for chemo-therapy), one of the resident physicians asked if I was from Chamberlain. He said that the Stroger staff and physicians have discussed how "Chamberlain treats the students like family." The young resident said, "As a student, I have needed someone to care for me and wish I had that type of experience in my learning environment." From Deb Tauber helping Phil to the car upon his last discharge, to the International Team calling Phil and checking on him, to our lab team setting up the testing environment for Phil to take the first HESI in the hospital bed, to our CAS doing remediation via conference and study packets, to his capstone faculty sending his assignments to his home...on and on. As we left his bedside today, I realized that our roles are so important to the lives of so many—we have many opportunities to make a difference every moment of every day. I am humbled to work for an organization that truly walks the walk.

OPERATIONALIZING CARE FOR PRELICENSURE STUDENTS

The Initial Pilot

Introduced in Chapter 2, Chamberlain developed a model (see Figure 2.1) to opera-tionalize *Chamberlain Care* based on the student life cycle. The operationalization of *Chamberlain Care* gave us the foundation for addressing critical touchpoints in the life cycle.

Chamberlain's ultimate objective was to achieve best-in-class student outcomes, and to differentiate Chamberlain through a culture of care and service. Specifically, the goal was to provide Chamberlain students with support, caring, and nurturing aimed at helping them succeed to learn, matriculate, graduate, pass the national nursing licens-ing exam (NCLEX-RN), gain employment, and be empowered to provide extraordinary care to people and families.

Planning Phase

After conducting the prelicensure BSN cohort retention study in spring 2012 that showed 28 percent of students are lost in the first five semesters, the *Chamberlain Care* Steering Council established a task force to develop a pilot study. The pilot focused on the first nursing course in the prelicensure curriculum—NR-101, Transitions to Nursing—with a goal of making an impact on student retention in the first year of the curriculum.

There were several data points that guided our focus on the first nursing course. First was the data that Chamberlain collected from course and faculty end-of-course evaluations, as well as classroom observations of faculty. The data indicated that stu-dents were disengaged and dissatisfied with the course; many thought the course con-sisted of busy work that was irrelevant to their nursing program. Faculty placed primary emphasis on American Psychological Association (APA) format and study skills that most students believed they had learned in other college courses. Second, we discovered that faculty did not enjoy the course because of the subject matter and therefore likely disengaged in their own ways.

As we addressed the opportunities in teaching this course, we made two decisions. First, the course was an ideal opportunity to introduce and evoke enthusiasm about nursing and becoming an extraordinary nurse. Students came to our program to become nurses and had high expectations for their first nursing course after being in general education courses. Second, the best strategy for heightening enthusiasm for the course was to use more engaging teaching-learning strategies and provide content that inspired enthusiasm about nursing and the student's role in it. Additionally, our assumption was that by enhancing student engagement early in the program, we could make a positive impact on retention early on.

There is a burgeoning body of literature supporting active teaching-learning strategies like those mentioned earlier that we promoted as part of *Chamberlain Care.* Active learning requires engaged, caring faculty willing to embrace pedagogies beyond the traditional ones that many learned in their own programs. The benefits of active learning extend beyond academic success (Everly, 2013) and student retention (Blessinger & Winkel, 2012) to improving practice development (Bakon, Craft, Christensen, & Wirihana, 2016; Dewing, 2010) in nursing students. Active learning was the antidote we needed to create a learning environment focused on care for the student, because it provides the context for students to engage in the material through reading, writing, talking, listening, and reflecting. The benefits of engagement through innovative activities include improved critical thinking skills, increased retention and transfer of new information, increased motivation, and improved interpersonal skills (Carpenter, Reddix, & Martin, 2016; Crookes, Crookes, & Walsh, 2013; Lucas, Testman, Hoyland, Kimble, & Euler, 2013). One of the important messages we conveyed in helping faculty appreciate the power of active learning was that the techniques enhance the retention of knowledge. The integration of active learning strategies as part of *Chamberlain Care* was built on Ken Bain's groundbreaking work, *What the Best College Teachers Do* (2004), which led to the teaching excellence training embodied in *Master Instruction* fully described in Chapter 3.

The pilot task force was comprised of some of our best and most innovative faculty charged with redesigning the first nursing course, Transitions in Nursing, to be more engaging, teach students coping and study skills, and connect students to their reasons for wanting to be a nurse. There were several goals of the course revision:

1. Shift the focus from rote memorization of principles to self-awareness, self-reflection, and accountability.

2. Review the course flow to reflect the continuum from successful person to successful student to successful professional nurse.

3. Incorporate a learning agreement between the students and faculty to emphasize the student's responsibility in the learning process.

4. Replace the content-laden lectures with experiential learning activities taught by faculty who were skilled at strategies that foster engagement and deep learning (named by Chamberlain as *Master Instruction*). These faculty adopted

the philosophy and principles outlined in Ken Bain's book, *What the Best College Teachers Do* (2004), mentioned previously.

5. We converted the classroom lectures into self-directed success seminars that students take virtually or in the Chamberlain Center for Academic Success (CAS) on each campus. We implemented nine online success seminars specific to the student that help introduce students to the professional nurse continuum. We also developed success seminars that students requested, including the topics of time management, study skills, anatomy and physiology, and medical terminology. We required students to take at least three of the seminars during the course—of their own choosing. Students received credit for taking the seminars.

We believe that students who avail themselves of the vast support resources we have available through our Centers for Academic Success tend to do better in the program than students who do not take advantage of resources. To that end, we required students (through a treasure hunt for which they received points in the course) to find and use college resources on their own initiative, such as the library and the CAS. The course content and structure was revised in May 2012 to reflect the goals discussed earlier. The decision to focus the pilot and major continuous improvement projects on student retention required buy-in and commitment of all Chamberlain leaders and faculty and staff. A series of meetings was scheduled for sharing the vision of *Chamberlain Care* and the specifics of the pilot. The pilot was launched at two campuses in July 2012. After observing statistically significant results in retention on those two campuses, the pilot was expanded to two other campuses in March 2013. Modifications to the course were made based on student and faculty feedback and evaluation. The initiative was expanded to all campuses in September 2013.

Measuring the Results of the Pilot

Various measures were used to evaluate the effectiveness of the pilot, including faculty and student satisfaction with the course, student and faculty perceptions of student self-efficacy at the end of the course, retention of pilot students from NR-101 to the next session compared to control campuses, and student performance in NR-224, Fundamentals-Skills, the next nursing course that traditionally has a high number of failures. Pilot outcomes specific to these measures are discussed next.

Student Satisfaction with NR-101. End-of-course survey satisfaction results for NR-101 averaged 3.33 on a four-point scale (September 2012 to July 2013) for all campuses except the four pilot campuses ($n = 650$), and 3.54 post pilot (September 2013 to January 2014) for all campuses except for the pilot campuses ($n = 909$), showing a statistically significant increase in end-of-course student satisfaction with NR-101 ($p < .001$).

Student Retention. As shown in Figures 4.1 and 4.2, tracking at the end of each semester showed that the pilot NR-101 cohorts on two campuses surpassed overall Chamberlain retention. Retention on one campus, which was already quite high, decreased slightly

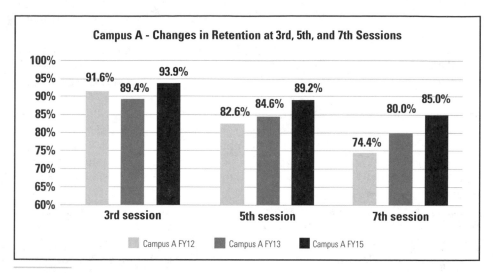

FIGURE 4.1 Comparing fiscal years (FY) 2012, 2013, and 2015 cohort retention for Campus A. Note: Chamberlain teaches its curriculum in 8-week increments called *sessions*. Two 8-week sessions equal one semester. Third-session retention reflects students continuously enrolled between Semesters 1 and 2; 5th-session retention indicates students who continue from Semester 2 to Semester 3, and 7th-session shows retention from Semester 3 to Semester 4. There are no summer breaks. Students are continuously enrolled for 9 semesters, completed year-round in 3 years. The average student transfers in at least 12 college credits and completes the program in 2½ years. NR-101 is the first nursing course, taught in Session 3 for students who have no transfer credit. Note: Chamberlain's fiscal year is July 1–June 30.

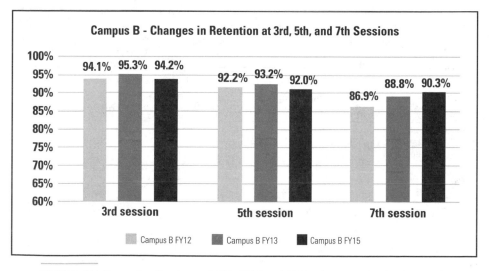

FIGURE 4.2 Comparing fiscal years 2012, 2013, and 2015 cohort retention for Campus B.

from fiscal year (FY) 2012 to FY 2013 but remained significantly higher than the Chamberlain overall average at that time.

Retention on Campus A slightly decreased for the third session for FY 2013 cohorts (but still was greater than the average of all campuses for FY 2013 cohorts), but retention increased at the fifth and seventh sessions for FY 2013 cohorts compared to FY 2012 cohorts. For Campus A, overall retention declined 17.2 percentage points from the third to seventh sessions for FY 2012 cohorts (pre-*Chamberlain Care*), but decline was less for FY 2013 cohorts (9.4 percentage points).

Comparing pre-*Chamberlain Care* to the most current fiscal year for which we have data through the seventh session, improvements in retention are more dramatic. Overall retention on Campus A declined 8.9 percentage points from the third to seventh sessions for FY 2015 cohorts.

Retention on Campus B showed slight improvement at each session. Overall retention declined 7.2 percentage points for FY 2012 cohorts with a smaller decline of 6.5 percentage points for FY 2013 cohorts and 3.9 percentage points for FY 2015 cohorts. Although Campus B did not show the significant percentage point change realized by Campus A each year, it is noteworthy that the overall retention rates for Campus B improved year to year for the seventh session (86.9 percent in FY 2012 compared to 90.3 percent in FY 2015).

Although we have not reached the 5-year retention goals established in FY 2012, we did make progress. At the time of the pilot, NR-101 was a one-credit-hour course. In FY 2016, the course was expanded to be two credit hours and is now standard fare for all students. We cannot say for certain that the changes we made to the first nursing course caused the retention improvements, but we do believe that the changes have had an impact on student success. We helped set student expectations of accountability; changed the attitude and expectations of the faculty; engaged students in the classroom; and through interactive and meaningful assignments, connected students early with resources that helped them succeed, taught them success strategies, and showed them that we care about their success. The model provided the framework for the concrete acts necessary for our quality improvement initiatives to improve student success.

Student Success in Subsequent Courses. After the pilot on the original two campuses, students were evaluated for their success in courses further along in their curriculum to determine whether the change in teaching-learning strategies or other factors affected their success. Grade distributions were evaluated in the next nursing course (NR-224, Fundamentals of Nursing Practice), which had a high failure rate on these two campuses prior to the pilot. This is the first major nursing course and generally requires students to think in a completely different way than what they have been accustomed to in previous academic studies. Students shift from rote memorization of content to a heavy emphasis on critical thinking, synthesis of material, and responding to NCLEX-RN–style questions on assessments. The results from those taking the NR-224 course comparing the session prior to pilot implementation (235 course takers) to the session a year after implementation (298 course takers) showed the following grade distribution results:

> The percent of A's and B's increased from 48 to 73 percent
> The percent of C's decreased from 37 to 20 percent
> The percent of failures and withdrawals decreased from 15 to 7 percent.

Although this was not a controlled study, we believe that early introduction to support resources and experientially-based teaching-learning strategies improved both retention and success.

In addition to tracking specific metrics, the task force continued to meet and identify lessons learned that could be applied for continuous improvement of that course and other courses in the curriculum. Over the course of the next several years, the same strategies and principles were integrated into all courses in the undergraduate and graduate curricula as part of the *Master Instruction* initiative described in Chapter 3.

Prelicensure Student Success Strategies Beyond the Pilot

Courses are only one aspect of how we interact with students, albeit a critical one. We subsequently engaged the entire college in initiatives to have a broader impact, and to achieve the overall culture we desired. The following are some examples of initiatives that have focused on various aspects of the student life cycle.

Individualized Student Support: The Chamberlain Care Student Success Model

Elements of the pilot to improve student retention were combined in a comprehensive model for prelicensure BSN student success that became known as the *Chamberlain Care* Student Success Model (CCSSM). The CCSSM is a fully integrated, holistic model of student support that exemplifies Chamberlain's commitment to provide prelicensure students extraordinary academic and nonacademic support that leads to exemplary learning outcomes, success on the professional licensing exam, and positive transition to a postgraduation role. The CCSSM incorporates a holistic approach to student academic support by focusing on critical moments throughout the life cycle of the student prior to admission through postgraduation. The model provides guidance in the use of standardized nationally normed assessments and provision of approaches and resources based on individual student and cohort needs across 20 campuses.

The CCSSM can be summarized as consisting of three primary components: student life cycle risk assessments, individualized student support, and NCLEX-RN preparation.

Life Cycle Risk Assessments: Chamberlain Early Assessment Program

The key to successful *early* identification, categorization, and success planning is the first level of assessment. Realizing that both academic and nonacademic factors influence a student's success, Chamberlain developed the Chamberlain Early Assessment Program (CEAP), a comprehensive assessment of academic and nonacademic factors that are strongly associated with students' potential for academic success and retention in their nursing program. The CEAP was developed from two primary sources, the Nurse Resilience Survey, a tool developed by Linda Hollinger-Smith (2017), who has a manuscript in preparation, and the Motivated Strategies for Learning Questionnaire (MSLQ) (Pintrich & DeGroot, 1990).

The Nurse Resilience Survey was constructed from a review of the literature and research on characteristics of resilience among nurses. Some of these factors associated with resilience addressed in the instrument include level of stress (Chesak et al., 2015), social support (Wang, Tao, Brown, & Zhang, 2017), being goal focused (Hart, Brannan, & De Chesnay, 2014), and demonstrating self-regulation of emotions (Grant & Kinman, 2013). Reliability, validity, and analysis of the factor analytic structure of the Nurse Resilience Survey scales were conducted, showing good internal consistency and convergent validity with other measures of resilience.

The MSLQ was developed to examine use of learning strategies and motivation among college students (Pintrich & DeGroot, 1990). Available in the public domain, the instrument has been used widely, and reliability and predictive validity have been reported (Pintrich, Smith, Garcia, & McKeachie, 1993; Cook, Thompson, & Thomas, 2011). Items from the MSLQ focusing on students' critical thinking abilities, motivation, learning beliefs, abilities to integrate new and existing knowledge, and comfort with peer learning experiences were part of the CEAP survey. Additional items identified in the literature associated with nursing student success were also included in the CEAP survey. Some of these factors included students' level of self-confidence and commitment (Dempsey & Reilly, 2016), sense of belonging (Liljedahl, Bjorck, Kalen, Ponzer, & Laksov, 2016), self-directed learning (Kan'an & Osman, 2015), and ability to balance work and school responsibilities (Silvestri, Clark, & Moonie, 2013). Initial psychometric testing of the CEAP survey scales with a sample of 2,435 nursing students showed good internal consistency reliability. A factor analysis was conducted to establish construct validity. Orthogonal varimax rotation identified 18 factors (cutoff point eigenvalue > 1.0) accumulatively explaining 59.2 percent of the variance.

The CEAP is administered online in class during the students' first nursing course. CEAP components are reassessed annually so that campus leadership may better understand the impact of the CCSSM on students' psychosocial factors, learning strategies, and motivation toward academic success and persistence over the course of their program, as well as evaluate potential differences among subgroups of students to better individualize program interventions. Chamberlain's Office of Institutional Effectiveness and Research closely tracks each student cohort participating in the CCSSM to evaluate the impact of CEAP results on retention and NCLEX-RN results.

Results of the CEAP assessment are provided to each campus and individually to each student via unique student reports (one for each student), and an aggregate campus-level report is provided to campus leadership. Included in student and advisor reports are hyperlinks to suggested "focused activities" associated with each topic area assessed in the CEAP. The focused activities are specific to the areas of student risk of dropping out or failure and are meant to be used by students to remediate risks. Some areas of student risk, rationale of importance to student success, and examples of focused activities are provided in Table 4.1.

Students who are identified as "at risk" in any of the risk categories are assigned activities designed to ameliorate the risk. Focused activities are considered "stepping stones" to help students understand what is important for their success and provide opportunities for students and advisors to discuss how nonacademic factors may influence student success in the nursing program. These are opportunities to empower the student with the knowledge and an introduction to tools to help them address these key areas.

TABLE 4.1

Focused Activities to Moderate Student Risk as Identified on CEAP Assessment

Area of Student Risk/Rationale	Example Focused Activity
Ability to focus on and commit to goals; setting short- and long-term goals are important skills needed to succeed in the nursing program and in one's nursing career to provide excellent care to patients	Identify a goal to accomplish with a career in nursing; formulate a SMART(ER) (specific, measurable, achievable, realistic, time specific) goal; work through the SMART steps to formulate a plan to accomplish the goal
Critical thinking and problem solving skills; critical thinking skills necessary in performing a nursing assessment, intervention, or acting as a patient advocate to prioritize and problem solve	Identify critical thinking skills that are strengths and those that are opportunities to work on; work through an exercise to test critical thinking abilities
Time management skills; increase awareness of how one organizes one's time, and plan good study skills	Students watch a video to learn time management tips and skills and are directed to work with their advisor on applying learning to develop good study habits
Building one's self-confidence; one of the most influential factors impacting learning, goal setting, and sense of commitment	Exercise to help develop positive core beliefs and a positive self-image and reinforce positive self-talk

A beginning student on the Sacramento campus commented during a student focus group that her CEAP assessment showed she was at risk because she was not engaged in the campus community and tended to stay by herself:

I realized I could either fade into the background and risk failing or I could get my butt in gear and get involved in my campus. I tend to be reserved, but I noticed that the environment at Chamberlain is not competitive like it is at other nursing schools where people are vying for seats. At Chamberlain, students help each other. It's like a family. I joined the student government association and took a part-time job as a student worker in the Center for Academic Success. Not only am I more involved in my campus, I'm doing better in school. I am grateful for the CEAP assessment, because it's nothing I would have recognized without having the results in black and white. But even then, you have to be willing to do something with the results.

Other Assessments. Standardized, nationally normed assessments are conducted throughout the program to determine knowledge gaps and guide the development of a personalized support plan to bridge the gaps.

Personalized Support Plan

The second major element of the CCSSM is individualized student support. Colleagues from academics, student services, and centers for academic success on each campus collaborate to develop an individualized support plan for each student based on a variety of assessments and key academic performance data. Mentoring, tutoring, and coaching is tailored to the student's needs. As the student progresses through the program assessments, academic performance data are monitored and used to modify the plan through the student life cycle. A CCSSM scorecard was developed to encapsulate results of assessments (see later discussion). The CCSSM scorecard aligns with critical touchpoints in the life cycle of the student. In addition, a tracking tool was developed that provides results in each subdomain for each student. Faculty and student advisors use this tool to track focused activities completed. They use the results from the tracking tool for student meetings to discuss progress. CEAP survey items are repeated for each student in Year 2 and Year 3 of the program to assess progress in these important nonacademic areas that impact student success.

NCLEX-RN Success

Instilling students with a culture of success on the NCLEX begins when the student is first admitted and continues throughout the entire curriculum. During the final capstone course, the student completes a comprehensive predictor assessment, which is predictive of NCLEX-RN success. The predictor assessment provides the student with an individualized plan and resources or remediation designed to address the student's individual learning gaps. A virtual tutor works directly with each student, using results from modular assessments to promote remediation and ultimate NCLEX-RN success.

At the end of the capstone course, each student is provided a comprehensive assessment to guide additional study in preparation for taking NCLEX-RN. Graduates of the prelicensure BSN are offered the opportunity to continue to work with mentors and tutors after graduation to ensure readiness for the NCLEX-RN. This includes virtual webinars, virtual tutoring sessions, phone contact for review and support, and use of electronic chat and cell phone texts up to the day the student sits for the licensure examination. Some campuses have tailored these approaches further and invited alumni to participate as mentors, and have arranged for faculty to meet students off campus to accommodate schedules and travel in more urban areas.

Our national academic success team surveys students to help evaluate the perceived value of our CCSSM approaches when they conduct a live review on a campus.

Student comment exemplifying the typical response to the support resources provided to students:

> I am thankful to be at a school that genuinely cares for my success. It is helpful to know early on my strengths and weaknesses in terms of the NCLEX. It was helpful to get material I can carry on to prepare for my NCLEX-RN as well as learning test taking strategies that I can use through the remainder of my program.

USING DATA TO DRIVE EVIDENCE-BASED DECISIONS

Tracking and Predicting Prelicensure Program Outcomes

Embarking on a plan to track and assess outcomes of *Chamberlain Care* for students required a fresh approach to program evaluation. The methodology selected addresses the impact of interventions at critical points in the program, provides reliable feedback to campus leaders and faculty informing the continued development of a caring culture for students, and predicts the probability of each student's propensity to succeed. Additionally, the program evaluation needed to take a comprehensive approach in assessing both academic and nonacademic factors associated with care for students and recognizing those key factors driving student success.

This section introduces the use of propensity modeling as an approach to evaluate the likelihood of academic success at given points in the student's program to apply interventions as early as possible to improve student outcomes. To better understand and address predictors of student success, a propensity model was developed for the prelicensure BSN program. Eventually, propensity modeling will be designed and employed across postlicensure programs as well.

Predictors of Prelicensure Nursing Student Success

Predicting outcomes of prelicensure BSN nursing student success, particularly on NCLEX-RN, has been an important focus of nursing programs for more than 30 years. With the continued national nursing shortages, the need to increase numbers of nurses from varied cultural backgrounds to meet the health care needs of an increasingly diverse population, and emphasis on first-attempt NCLEX-RN pass rates as a crucial measure of student achievement, the need to take a proactive approach to predict success outcomes across the program of study is paramount.

The process of identifying prospective predictors of student success at Chamberlain began with an extensive review of the research literature. There are several potential student success outcomes previously studied in the literature, including first-semester performance (Kowitlawakul, Brenkus, & Dugan, 2012), end-of-program GPA performance (Cunningham, Manier, Anderson, & Sarnosky, 2014), results of standardized testing (Wolkowitz & Kelley, 2010), and student retention rates (Bigbee & Mixon, 2013).

Factors predicting prelicensure student success on the NCLEX-RN may be categorized as academic or nonacademic. Examples of academic predictors of NCLEX-RN success identified in the literature include HESI Admission Assessments (A2) (Hinderer, DiBartolo, & Walsh, 2014), preadmission cumulative GPA (Hopkins, 2008), Scholastic Aptitude Test (SAT) scores (Haas, Nugent, & Rule, 2004), prerequisite science GPA (Bentley, 2006), standardized achievement tests taken during the program of study (Chen, Heiny, & Lin, 2014), standardized exit examinations (Nibert & Young, 2001), and higher GPAs in nursing courses (Romeo, 2013).

Fewer studies have examined nonacademic predictors of prelicensure student success on the NCLEX-RN examination. Hopkins (2008) found associations between NCLEX-RN success and critical thinking abilities, learning style, degree of commitment, level of anxiety, age, ethnic background, and gender among senior generic nursing students. Romeo's study (2013) of the relationship between critical thinking skills and NCLEX-RN success further supported the contention that critical thinking, particularly goal setting ability, is a significant predictor of NCLEX-RN success.

Findings of many studies exploring academic and nonacademic predictors of NCLEX-RN have been inconclusive at best due to methodologic issues such as small sample sizes, differences in metrics used, and diversity of students across nursing programs. Chamberlain has engaged in studies using our own student data to inform decision making and student support initiatives.

Chamberlain Studies of Key Predictors of Prelicensure Student Success. Conducting nationwide studies of NCLEX-RN predictors across the multiple Chamberlain campuses allowed the opportunity to address several of the issues inherent in previous studies.

Chamberlain's studies focused on identifying key academic factors, both preadmission and nursing program related, predictive of student success on the NCLEX-RN examination. The target population included all prelicensure BSN students who tested from July 2013 through September 2015. Supporting findings from earlier studies (Kaddoura, Flint, Van Dyke, Yang, & Chiang, 2016), Chamberlain students with previous baccalaureate degrees had higher pass rates compared to those with previous associate degrees. Similar to previous studies (McGahee, Gramling, & Reid, 2010; Hopkins, 2008), higher NCLEX-RN pass rates were found among Chamberlain students with greater high school GPAs and those from Caucasian backgrounds. There were no differences between Chamberlain students who passed or failed based on age, gender, parents' education, or number of years since completion of high school.

Students who took their prerequisite science courses (i.e., Introduction to Chemistry, Microbiology, and Anatomy & Physiology) at Chamberlain had higher NCLEX-RN pass rates compared to those transferring one or more science courses. We suspect that this finding may be explained by the recency of prerequisite science courses taken at Chamberlain compared to those transferred as well as the greater variability among courses transferred to Chamberlain. This second explanation is further supported by the finding that the greater the number of prerequisite science courses transferred to Chamberlain, the lower the NCLEX-RN pass rates.

Standardized preadmission testing in topic areas including English vocabulary, reading comprehension, sciences, and mathematics is required of all Chamberlain prelicensure BSN applicants. All individual preadmission assessment scores were significantly greater for students passing NCLEX-RN compared to those failing, with the greatest difference between these groups noted for vocabulary scores.

To understand to what degree individual preadmission assessments predicted NCLEX-RN results, a stepwise regression model was constructed identifying the effect size for each individual assessment in relation to NCLEX-RN findings. The individual assessments found to have the greatest effect on NCLEX-RN results were (in order of greatest to lesser effects) vocabulary, reading comprehension, biology, and anatomy and physiology. As a result of this analysis, a custom composite score was built as a key tool used in admissions decision making.

Similar to many nursing colleges, Chamberlain has identified key metrics and scoring ranges that serve as a guide assisting prelicensure BSN campus admission committees in the assessment of the quality of prelicensure applicants. These metrics are combined in the form of an admission matrix developed to provide a useful data point to assist in the admission process.

The purpose of the second study was to validate scoring ranges and weightings for a new admission matrix scoring system. The target population included the September 2015 starting cohort of students who had admission decision reports. A new admission matrix score was calculated for each September 2015 applicant, with results validated against the actual admission decisions. Differences among the new admission matrix scores compared to the three categories of actual admission decisions (i.e., academically eligible, accepted provisionally, and rejected) were highly significant ($p < .001$), indicating that the new admission matrix scoring differentiates among admission decision categories in the desired direction.

Additionally, the validation study results supported the need to revise transfer credit policies in relation to both prerequisite science courses and nursing courses taken at other colleges. The transfer credit policy related to prerequisite science courses was revised such that a grade of C would transfer only if the corresponding first-time preadmission assessment score on that science content was 72 or greater. If the corresponding preadmission assessment score was below 72 for that particular transfer science course in which a grade of C was earned, that science course must be repeated or advanced placement test passed successfully.

Study results confirmed that the percentage of students failing NCLEX-RN was greatest for those transferring in C grades from foundational nursing courses (i.e., pathophysiology, pharmacology, and nutrition), particularly if the courses were taken at 2-year community colleges. The transfer credit policy related to nursing courses was revised as a result of these findings to require that nursing courses accepted for transfer be completed with a grade of B or better from a course deemed acceptable in a baccalaureate nursing program.

The application of a new admission matrix was a critical element in achieving the primary purpose of *Chamberlain Care* for students—admitting students with the propensity to succeed and providing the excellent services that would will help them achieve their goals and reach their dreams. As has been emphasized, this means improving retention that leads to graduation and NCLEX-RN success for our prelicensure students. The research we conducted allowed us to differentiate more precisely, based on the admission matrix components, which students are likely to stay in school and graduate. In refining our admission matrix to differentiate who is likely to succeed, we provide a service in line with *Chamberlain Care* that positions each applicant for potential success. It also allows us to leverage the academic success services to meet the needs of each cohort admitted in a more efficacious way.

Propensity Modeling: An Innovative Approach to Evaluate Likelihood of Students' Academic Success

One of the key challenges in educational research and measurement is the difficulty in designing methodologies that use randomization and demonstrate causal relationships (Montgomery, 2012). Students typically "self-select" into educational programs and class sections, making randomization highly unlikely due to practical and potentially ethical reasons. However, a good deal of educational research focuses on evaluating programs or interventions targeting improving student success outcomes. Nonexperimental methods using observations or correlations typically have been utilized in educational program evaluation, but neither is useful to establish causal effects or predict future outcomes.

What Is Propensity Modeling?

Propensity modeling is relatively new to educational research (Clark & Cundiff, 2011; Friedman & Mandel, 2009), having been primarily used in the field of economics. Fundamentally, propensity modeling is an analytical approach to reduce selection bias due to selecting samples that may not be representative of the population being studied, which is common in observational or nonexperimental research designs (Herzog, 2014). Through a series of multiple regression analyses, propensity modeling "balances" systematic differences to reduce systematic biases. Then "like" subjects are grouped according to a standardized propensity score based on the "best fit" among the regression models. For the propensity model to work best, the majority of factors that go into the model should be identified as predictive of the intended outcome. Identification of these factors can be both from the literature and from past studies.

Propensity modeling is an advanced form of multiple regression modeling that requires complex statistics expertise in application of statistical packages as well as access to large datasets of 5,000 or more student records. Smaller nursing programs may consider consulting with a statistician, who may recommend other techniques such as logistic regression or other forms of regression modeling for predictive analyses.

Chamberlain's Approach to Propensity Modeling

Chamberlain's focus on a culture of care to help students succeed in their program framed the approach taken to propensity modeling. This approach begins at preadmission and follows each student through the nursing program to the NCLEX-RN result. To that end, propensity modeling asks, "How likely is it for a student to succeed on the NCLEX-RN examination given results on specific factors (both academic and nonacademic) at given points in the nursing program?"

Unique to the propensity methodology is the ability to consider new assessment information for each student over the course of the program of study. A propensity score is calculated for each student at four key points of the program: (1) during the first nursing course, (2) at the end of Year 1, (3) at the end of Year 2, and (4) at the end of Year 3. From an advising perspective, using these key data points not only helps identify students who may be at risk earlier in the program but also allows faculty and advisors to track the impact of interventions in promoting student success.

Since the propensity modeling uses the maximum amount of information at a given point in the program to determine a student's score, any updated information in the modeling will update the student's propensity score. Figure 4.3 shows a diagram of the Chamberlain Propensity Model and key indicators entered into the propensity model at critical points of the program. Each propensity score critical point considers the key indicators for that particular program year in addition to all key indicators preceding that critical point. The "steps" of the model reflect the "additive" nature of the propensity model as the student progresses. It is important to note that other nursing programs may find that some key indicators predicting student success differ for their prelicensure BSN students. Diversity among nursing programs, applicant characteristics, admission criteria, and other factors influence selection of student success predictors.

The initial propensity score is derived from the custom preadmission composite score and previous high school/college cumulative GPAs. From Chamberlain's analysis of NCLEX-RN predictors, the custom preadmission composite score was the strongest early predictor of NCLEX-RN results measuring the most current aptitude for content areas including English vocabulary, reading comprehension, biology, and anatomy and physiology, all key content areas foundational to the nursing program. The Year 1 propensity score analysis includes key factors (academic and nonacademic) assessed during the students' first nursing course in addition to the total number of

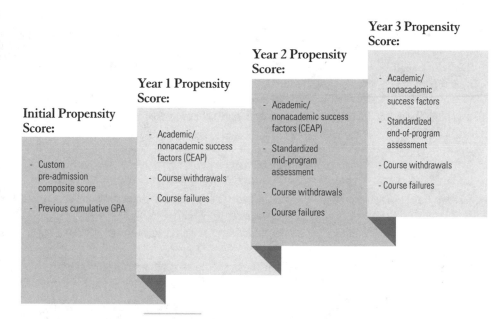

FIGURE 4.3 The Chamberlain Propensity Model.

course withdrawals and failures during the first year of the program. Based on assessment of the academic and nonacademic factors from the CEAP, two index scores are calculated: the Academic Success Index, indicating students' potential for academic success over the first year of the program, and the Retention Success Index, reflecting students' potential for retention into the following year.

Students are assessed annually on the nonacademic factors that may impact their potential for success and retention as they continue in their program. Some of these nonacademic factors identified in both the literature and Chamberlain's studies include self-confidence level, motivation for learning, social support network, degree of resilience, goal orientation, and sense of belonging. Chamberlain campuses have incorporated interventions based on these factors to empower students to become more self-confident, resilient, and goal-focused in their coursework. An example is shared later in this section.

Chamberlain prelicensure BSN students are also administered standardized nationally normed assessments during the course of their program. Years 2 and 3 propensity score analyses include results of these assessments in addition to ongoing evaluation of academic/nonacademic success factors and the total number of course withdrawals and failures during the second and third years of the program.

Strategies for Propensity Score Analysis

A CCSSM scorecard was developed to provide campus-, regional-, and national-level results on key indicators noted in the Chamberlain Propensity Model. Leaders may compare results semester to semester or year to year and track the progress of each new student cohort across the entire nursing program. Campus leaders also receive

TABLE 4.2

Example Implications and Findings From Propensity Model Key Indicators

Propensity Model Key Indicators	Implications/Findings Impacting Student Success
Custom preadmission composite score	• The custom preadmission composite score is the key preadmission driver of student success. • A composite score < 63 is high risk for NCLEX-RN failure; identify early remediation needs in English or science content.
Academic Success Index (CEAP)	• Identifies students by potential for academic success (i.e., high, moderate, low potential for success).
Retention Success Index (CEAP)	• Identifies students by potential to retain into Year 2 (i.e., high, moderate, low potential for success).
Number of course withdrawals and failures	• Average number of course withdrawals and failures for those failing NCLEX-RN is more than twice that of those passing NCLEX-RN. • For each year, content areas of courses in which students most often withdraw or fail and that are most associated with NCLEX-RN failure are targeted for remediation.
Standardized assessment examinations	• Identifies content areas in high and low academic risk zones for remediation via student success seminars. • Identify patterns in assessment results across cohorts.

Propensity score (PS)	• The end-of-program PS is highly correlated with NCLEX-RN results (following results based on nearly 1,000 graduates):
	  • NCLEX-RN pass rate of students at the high PS ranges was 96 percent.
	  • NCLEX-RN pass rate of students at the low PS ranges was 42 percent.

a detailed searchable spreadsheet of key indicators and propensity scores for each enrolled student to track and plan interventions for those at academic risk, empowering faculty, advisors, and students to take action as early as possible.

Table 4.2 provides some examples of implications and findings affecting student success derived from propensity model key indicators. Armed with information from Chamberlain studies showing the impact of key indicator results on student outcomes, faculty are empowered to design effective student success interventions.

Using Propensity Score Data to Design Student Success Interventions Supporting a Culture of Care

Chamberlain campuses develop student success interventions based on key indicator results identified in the propensity modeling. The addition of propensity scores in designing interventions was piloted at several campuses with positive results. Underlying these interventions is the focus on Chamberlain's culture of care, promoting student learning and engagement and fostering student–faculty relationship building.

From Leslie Pafford, PhD, RN, FNP-BC, president, Houston campus:

Good Morning Linda,

I just wanted to pause and be sure that I shared with you how appreciative I am of your work on the propensity model. It has made such a huge difference at our campus. Always wanting to base decisions on data, it got my attention when I first heard about it almost a year ago when you first began discussing this. Having the data available and looking at what it told us, we made needed changes in our program. We are seeing great success with our students and a climbing pass rate. Without the propensity model, we would be left hoping for positive outcomes instead of being able to take firm actions to assure success.

Thank you so much for your work on this. My team and I are very appreciative.

Applying Findings From Assessment of Nonacademic Success Indicators

Propensity modeling allows consideration of both academic and nonacademic factors that may impact student success. As discussed previously, nonacademic factors have been identified in both the literature and in Chamberlain studies as important predictors of student success. In Chamberlain's initial predictive model of factors driving NCLEX-RN results, only 26 percent of the variance was explained by academic factors. Few published studies separate the impact of academic and nonacademic factors on NCLEX-RN success. In one of the few previous studies to do so, Johnston (1990) found that 16 percent of the variance in NCLEX-RN results was explained by academic factors.

A student success intervention supporting the importance of nonacademic factors for student success was implemented in one of Chamberlain's early nursing courses focused on health and wellness. Faculty integrated key nonacademic concepts (resilience, motivation for learning, academic skills, learning strategies, etc.) into a self-care mapping experience for students to reflect and follow up on their interventions for self-care initially identified in the assessment completed in the first nursing course. The purpose of this activity is to emphasize for students that self-care is an important area for continued attention to support success during the program as a nursing student and beyond as a nursing professional.

Applying Findings From Assessment of Academic Success Indicators

Propensity data are being used by campuses to address academic issues experienced by students at various critical points in the program. Based on propensity scores, students at academic risk may be grouped to strategize interventions targeting their particular areas of weakness. This supports more efficient and effective use of tutoring resources, for example. Having propensity score information current at any point in the program has also resulted in campuses implementing remediation and assessments earlier in the program to better support readiness efforts for NCLEX-RN. Tracking each student cohort separately also has guided the development of individualized action plans for each cohort.

Propensity Modeling Next Steps

From a continuing quality improvement perspective, propensity modeling provides an effective methodology to derive meaning from large amounts of diverse data from multiple sources and to better understand the impact of Chamberlain services provided to students on vital outcome measures of student success—retain, learn, graduate, and pass NCLEX-RN.

Continued propensity modeling research will further Chamberlain's goals for its graduates by identifying key indicators predicting career success outcomes of Chamberlain alumni. Additionally, application of the predictive analysis approach, which is foundational to propensity modeling, is being applied to postlicensure programs, particularly in identifying factors predictive of student success in the family nurse practitioner program.

OPERATIONALIZING CARE FOR POSTLICENSURE STUDENTS

Although the Chamberlain postlicensure student might be attending any one of four different postlicensure or graduate nursing programs, the faculty and leadership identified similar characteristics in most students. The typical postlicensure student is a working adult nurse with significant job and family responsibilities who chooses online learning because of the ability to do the work anytime, anywhere, and in any situation. Most of the students have stressful jobs in clinical settings, often with leadership responsibilities, and many are caring for children and aging parents. These students have usually been out of school for several years, and they are anxious about adding the role and work of a student to a life that already seems too full. When asked about their motivation for returning to school, students typically give one of two reasons: (1) my employer requires it, or (2) I am doing this so I can secure a job or promotion. When asked what worries them most, they often answer that they are afraid they cannot find the time to do everything.

The educational and nursing literature support this understanding of postlicensure students' needs. Willging and Johnson (2009) reported that online graduate students most commonly reported leaving their online program because it was too difficult to carry a full-time job and do graduate work. Lee and Choi (2011) examined online program dropout rates and concluded that students' environmental challenges, such as work and personal commitments, had a significant effect on dropout decisions. A qualitative study by Perry, Boman, Care, Edwards, and Park (2008) found that the most common reason for withdrawing from an online graduate nursing program was an unexpected personal life event that eroded the availability of time, money, and energy. In a review of the graduate nursing and higher education literature, Gazza and Hunker (2014) found that helping postlicensure nursing students stay in school was a multifactorial challenge that required a multifactorial approach, including relationship building, providing quality programs and courses, and supporting students through challenging situations.

As part of our commitment to operationalizing *Chamberlain Care,* the Chamberlain leadership team asked the question, "What can we do to help anxious, busy, often overwhelmed students succeed and persist to graduation?" The team set a goal of increasing first-to-second session persistence in the RN-BSN program by one percentage point over the course of a year. They further established a subgoal to achieve a one percentage point persistence gain in each session compared to the same session in the previous year.

After several meetings and brainstorming sessions, the RN-BSN team settled on two strategies that focused on the student experience in the first course in the program, NR-351, Transitions to Professional Nursing:

▶ Assign one faculty manager to manage all sections of the first course, with no responsibilities for other courses.

▶ Create assignments in NR-351 to motivate students to complete the new student orientation and meet with a student service advisor.

For the first strategy, the RN-BSN leadership restructured the responsibilities of the faculty management team. At Chamberlain, the faculty managers oversee multiple courses, each with several sections. They are responsible for training and supporting the visiting professors (part-time or adjunct faculty) who teach most of the courses. As part of this initiative, the faculty manager over the first course in the program kept the supervision of only one course, NR-351, which had multiple sections, with no other responsibilities. An additional faculty manager was hired to lessen the burden of the other faculty managers in taking on additional courses. The idea was that if instructors teaching NR-351 were cared for by a dedicated faculty manager who was focused on their success, those instructors would then be able to give better care to their students. Having a single faculty manager responsible for a single course allowed the staff to respond to instructor needs and identify actual or potential problems more quickly, leading to more timely resolution and increased student satisfaction. The NR-351 faculty manager also developed a communication strategy for the course instructors, sending out regular updates and even sending birthday wishes to instructors. The dedicated NR-351 faculty manager was able to monitor instructor engagement more closely, and high-performing instructors were more easily identified for invitations to teach future NR-351 sections.

The second strategy was a collaborative effort between Chamberlain and DeVry Online Services (DOS), the organization that provides admissions, student services, course scheduling, and faculty operations support to Chamberlain. Historical anecdotal data suggested a correlation between (1) student participation in the new student orientation and meeting with a student service advisor and (2) increased first-session persistence. To further strengthen these student orientation processes, which were not mandatory, the faculty worked with course designers to improve the new student orientation, including material and activities about how to be successful in school, how to manage time, and how to use academic resources. The faculty then created several assignments in the first course that required student participation in the new student orientation and required students to attend a meeting with a student service advisor. As these changes were implemented, participation increased in both the new student orientation and the meetings with student service advisors.

The success of these initiatives in the RN-BSN program encouraged the other postlicensure programs to adopt them. In the years since the initial attempt, the faculty continued to improve the new student orientation and the program teams hired more faculty managers to support instructors in a focused and comprehensive manner. These initiatives have become standard operating procedure throughout the postlicensure programs, and the team has continued the process of identifying and developing ideas to show care for students.

Postlicensure Tracking of Student Outcomes

Tracking postlicensure student outcomes considers *Chamberlain Care* components including student retention, persistence, engagement, care from faculty, and excellence in service. Additionally, examples of *Chamberlain Care* that extend to postlicensure student mentors and preceptors are also evaluated during the course of the students' program. Including multiple perspectives from the lenses of the postlicensure student, faculty, mentors, and preceptors at key touchpoints provide valuable information to support student success within a caring culture.

Examples of Postlicensure Student Outcomes

Postlicensure retention into the students' second session is closely tracked for each program. A review of attrition rates from the past three fiscal years (2014 to 2016) revealed that the highest attrition rates in postlicensure online programs were found from the first session and into the second session of the programs. A target of 85 percent retention into the second session was chosen by leadership, and plans for addressing ways to improve retention were identified. Analysis of the DNP first-session courses revealed opportunities for interventions early in the program. DNP faculty reported that about a third of the students in each new DNP cohort struggled with academic writing. The faculty initiated a voluntary writing "boot camp" and offered it without cost to students. When students realized that they were in danger of failing their first DNP course because of poor writing, many decided to take advantage of the recommended tutoring. Boot camp students met with a writing instructor by phone and web several times a week to analyze their writing and make improvements.

Postlicensure session-to-session persistence is a measure of continuous student enrollment and is used to drive continuous quality improvement projects. Annual session-to-session persistence has remained stable across the postlicensure programs over the past three fiscal years (2015 to 2017), ranging from 82 to 88 percent.

Students are invited to complete an end-of-course survey each session. In addition to "typical" satisfaction measures related to courses, instructors, preceptors, and resources, the survey items also focus on metrics directly linked to *Chamberlain Care,* including student engagement, perceptions of care from faculty, and excellence in service.

A Student Engagement Index score, consisting of results from five items on the end-of-course survey, is assessed each semester. Postlicensure Student Engagement Index scores have consistently remained over the benchmark implemented in fiscal year 2014. Example student engagement items from the survey are as follows:

> I am assigned challenging tasks in this course that helped me think differently.

> This course promoted my curiosity to expand application of my learnings.

Students' perceptions of care from faculty are also measured at the end of each course. *Faculty caring* is defined as the degree of interest and helpful feedback perceived by students during their courses. Again, postlicensure students' perceptions of care from faculty are consistently above benchmarks since implementing this metric in fiscal year 2014.

As a measure of excellence in service, students are asked to respond at several points during each year of their program as to the degree they would recommend Chamberlain programs to other potential students. Using the tool *Net Promoter Score* (Satmetrix, 2017), a "promoter score" is calculated based on survey results and trends are tracked by each postlicensure program's leadership. When postlicensure faculty review the survey data and comments, they respond with ideas and an action plan for addressing students' concerns, often resulting in significant curricular changes or service improvement projects. For example, faculty in the MSN nonclinical specialty tracks became concerned about repeated comments from students regarding discontinuities in the final two courses in the program. A growing number of students said that they would not recommend the program to others because the last two courses contained repetitive projects and conflicting content. After digging into the courses from the students' perspective, faculty realized that they needed to redesign not only these courses but also the concluding practicum experience as a whole. Although the major changes required a 3-year implementation process, faculty made incremental improvements in the interim that addressed many of the students' concerns.

Chamberlain Care extends to postlicensure preceptors and mentors as well. After each clinical or mentoring experience, preceptors and mentors are asked to provide insights as to their experiences with Chamberlain students and faculty. In relationship to Chamberlain students, more than 90 percent of preceptors and mentors agreed or strongly agreed that students were well prepared, demonstrated competence in their performance, behaved professionally, and were open to constructive feedback. In regard to their experience with Chamberlain faculty, more than 90 percent of preceptors and mentors felt that expectations of their responsibilities were clearly defined, Chamberlain faculty were accessible, and student projects were consistent with the needs of their organizations. Additionally, the majority of preceptors and mentors felt that they learned new things about their own abilities, their experiences motivated them in their positions, and they would be likely to serve as a preceptor or mentor to a Chamberlain student in the future.

CHALLENGES AND OPPORTUNITIES OF CARE FOR STUDENTS
Prelicensure Students

The implementation of care for prelicensure BSN students has been an ongoing, intense, and comprehensive undertaking by Chamberlain that required attention to the holistic nature of academic preparation that builds on previous life experiences, engages the student in learning across a program cycle, leaves them with the knowledge and competencies for practice, and inspires them to engage in lifelong learning. However, the cornerstone of success where an educational institution has the most control is in retention. In a substantive review of the literature, Mooring (2016) examined emerging themes in research seeking to explicate challenges to nursing student retention and approaches to improve persistence. "The literature review supports the idea that poor retention is related not only to student ability, but also to a lack of necessary intervention by faculty beginning with the admission process and continuing throughout the curriculum"

(p. 204). This mirrors the conclusions at which we arrived that led to the development of *Chamberlain Care* and the CCSSM. Mooring concluded that alterations to support student retention need to be made at the level of recruitment and student selection and involve aggressive academic advising strategies, and that an overall retention program should be woven into the nursing curriculum.

Chamberlain Care and the CCSSM are the remedies for what we saw as outdated thinking about nursing education and academic preparation for practice. We faced the following challenges and opportunities:

1. ***Recruitment Practices and Admission Criteria:*** The challenge at Chamberlain was to achieve recruitment and admission of the most highly qualified individuals. We are committed to promoting diversity in health care and to supporting nontraditional students. By applying *Chamberlain Care* and knowledge from our analyses to our recruitment and admission process and standards, we were able to refine our admission criteria to capture those students that lie between the most qualified and those who are distinctly not qualified. By also identifying gaps in consistent application of admission criteria, we generated strategies to improve admission policies and practices.

2. ***Aggressive Advising as a Potential Solution:*** At Chamberlain, we recognized that there was compelling evidence in the literature in higher education on academic success that "intrusive advising" makes a difference. Our approach was to capitalize on the strong relationships that our student services and admissions advisors developed with students. Students often viewed these colleagues as their advocates. We view student support as a community endeavor involving advisors, academic faculty and leaders, and staff from our campus academic success centers. Aggressive, intentional advising was one component of a broader individualized approach that included elements of mentoring, coaching, and tutoring tailored at the discretion of campus leaders. Campus leaders were empowered to shape the broad approach into effective initiatives based on their culture, faculty, and student bodies.

   There were several major challenges encountered in launching and sustaining this new approach of aggressive, supportive advising. The first challenge was to clearly communicate the intent of the model to promote a positive perception of *Chamberlain Care* by the faculty, centers of academic success, and student advisors. We knew that they would be the crucial front line in gaining support from faculty, and ultimately students, for this new approach. This meant that the leaders in each of these areas had to communicate clearly the intent and expectations of *Chamberlain Care* to support the CCSSM and to clarify the type of relationship that we were promoting. It required knowing the behaviors associated with care, building them into performance reviews, and hiring new colleagues who demonstrated these behaviors. It also meant believing in an educational culture of empowering and emboldening students. We created a comprehensive training program detailed previously to ensure that new and continuing colleagues learned to apply *Chamberlain Care* effectively and would continue to develop their strengths throughout their work life with us.

   The second challenge was changing student perceptions of what *Chamberlain Care* student support meant. We accomplished this in part by the changes we made in the orientation to include *Chamberlain Care* and the CCSSM, re-emphasizing it in the first nursing course that focused on engaged student learning and getting students to agree to meet certain expectations for assignments. Just as with faculty, we were required to remind students in critical conversations the difference between enabling, which would not be successful, and empowering through *Chamberlain Care.*

The third challenge was promoting a new form of faculty–student rapport that would create the caring student–faculty relationships. Since faculty are in the most direct contact with students, this relationship was at the heart of transforming the culture of Chamberlain. Finding the balance of building a professional relationship that promotes learning while personalizing the educational experience for a student has always been a challenge. Launching the *Chamberlain Care* initiative helped us appreciate how important it was to engage faculty in conversations on the meaning of teaching and learning in a culture of care. We were heartened to learn that most of our faculty actually yearned for new and more engaging approaches to the student–teacher experience that would enable them to unleash the greatest potential of the student. We started with advocates and exemplary faculty, who became a central resource on each campus. We provided annual awards to recognize faculty and other colleagues who embodied *Chamberlain Care* in their work with students.

3. ***Retention Programs Woven Into the Curriculum:*** We knew that to be successful, *Chamberlain Care* and the CCSSM must be woven into the curriculum and throughout every aspect of the student experience. The greatest challenge of this integration was the sheer comprehensiveness of the program; the scope of reach of our campuses; and, most importantly, our desire for a full cultural transformation. The ability to generate and analyze data to demonstrate the need for change and engender faith in the approaches built into the CCSSM enhanced buy-in of colleagues. Curriculum changes are never simple, and revising learning outcomes and adding and changing requirements and assignments proved onerous. To make these changes effectively, we relied on our process of governance and used leaders to foster review and approval for changes. A signature aspect of our governance process is that curricular change proposals are submitted with specific rationale and evidence to support the change using a standard format. Once proposals are presented, there is a 30-day period for comment. This approach allows for important feedback and engenders greater support among faculty and leaders. Chamberlain uses national teams of academic success, clinical education, curriculum, and faculty development/training experts for the prelicensure BSN program. These experts, along with their leaders, helped ensure the transition to new ways of approaching teaching-learning and supporting academic success.

Postlicensure Students

Much of the literature on graduate student success in online programs emphasizes the importance of strong relationships between faculty and students (Lee & Choi, 2011; Gazza & Hunker, 2014). Building relationships in a large postlicensure online program is challenging and requires an intentional approach. The postlicensure leadership and faculty are focusing their efforts on the following new initiatives, which are showing early signs of success:

1. ***Voluntary Synchronous Faculty/Student Meetings:*** Although online students famously want completely asynchronous requirements so that they can do their work at any time of the day or night, a significant number seem to benefit from the opportunity to interact "in person." In the distance environment, this means offering a web-based option for audio and visual interactions through microphones and cameras. As an experiment, the RN-BSN faculty began offering synchronous web-based "Meet and Greets" to students early in the first course. To their surprise, more than 30 percent of the new students attended the initial meetings, and the attendance numbers have continued to grow. Students use the time to ask questions, hear from faculty and leadership, and connect with the community of their peers. This initiative opened a communication door that created more interactions between faculty and students—interactions that continued by email and phone after the webinar. Early results indicate a significant impact on first-session persistence as well. The postlicensure team is evaluating this effort for implementation in other programs.

2. ***Increased Email and Phone Touchpoints:*** Faculty in all programs are reaching out to students more frequently through email and phone. The purpose of the outreach is to express care for students. Faculty are sending birthday greetings, asking how things are going, and offering their assistance. The reports from this kind of outreach are encouraging. Students often express surprise that a faculty member would make a personal contact unrelated to a course assignment. Sometimes faculty learn about special challenges that a student is facing— things the student would not have shared with the instructor without prompting. Learning about these challenges allows faculty to give additional support.

3. ***Flexibility in Assignment Deadlines:*** As faculty hear more from students through increased interactions, they learn about pain points. Students report that strict assignment deadlines with high penalties are very discouraging to them. They would like to see more flexibility in accepting completed assignments to accommodate the nurse who might have to work ten 12-hour shifts in a row while caring for children and a sick parent. This is a struggle for faculty, who must balance their own deadlines for grading assignments and submitting course grades. Recent discussions have centered on how to support students facing unusual challenges while maintaining fair expectations. The culture of care is a centerpiece of these discussions, and faculty often remark on how much they appreciate the support, help, and forgiveness of deadlines that they have received from leadership and colleagues amid a difficult personal situation. They want to transmit this care to students without compromising the educational work that must occur. The faculty is piloting revised assignment deadline guidelines toward that end.

Building a caring community in an online program requires thoughtful, intentional interventions built on student input. Every piece of the program needs to make students' lives easier, not more difficult, as much as that is possible within the demands of academic achievement. The postlicensure programs team envisions a future where students can do their best work because they are relieved of unnecessary demands and irrelevant activities. Striving to achieve that future motivates the team to participate in constant evaluation and continuous improvement.

References

Bain, K. (2004). *What the best college teachers do.* Cambridge, MA: Harvard University Press.

Bakon, S., Craft, J., Christensen, M., & Wirihana, L. (2016). Can active learning principles be applied to the bioscience assessment of nursing students? A review of the literature. *Nursing Education Today, 37,* 123–127. doi:10.1016/j.nedt.2015.11.030

Bankert, E. G., & Kozel, V. (2005). Transforming pedagogy in nursing education: A caring learning environment for adult students. *Nursing Education Perspectives, 26*(4), 227–229.

Beck, C. T. (2001). Caring within nursing education: A metasynthesis. *Journal of Nursing Education, 40*(3), 101–109. doi:10.3928/0148-4834-20010301-04

Bentley, R. (2006). Comparison of traditional and accelerated baccalaureate nursing graduates. *Nurse Educator, 31*(2), 79–83. Available at http://www.nursingcenter.com/journalarticle?Article_ID=648220

Bigbee, J., & Mixon, D. (2013). Recruitment and retention of rural nursing students: A retrospective study. *Rural and Remote Health, 13*(4), 2486–2488. Available at https://www.ncbi.nlm.nih.gov/pubmed/24160687

Blessinger, P., & Winkel, L. A. (2012). *Increasing student engagement and retention using immersive interfaces: Virtual worlds, gaming, and simulation.* Bingley, UK: Emerald Group Publishing.

Carpenter, S., Reddix, R., & Martin, D. (2016). Pills, thrills, and pharmacology drills! Strategies to increase student retention in an entry-level nursing pharmacology course. *Teaching and Learning in Nursing, 11,* 179–183. doi:10.1016/j.teln.2016.04.002

Chamberlain University College of Nursing. (2017). *Chamberlain College of Nursing Academic Catalog 2017–2018.* Retrieved from http://www.chamberlain.edu/docs/default-source/academics-admissions/chp-catalog.pdf?sfvrsn=8

Chen, H., Heiny, E. L., & Lin, C. (2014). Development of a prediction model for early diagnosis of not passing the National Council of Licensure Examination for registered associated degree nurses. *Studies in Health Technology and Informatics, 201,* 271–276.

Chesak, S. S., Bhagra, A., Schroeder D. R., Foy, D. A., Cutshall, S. M., & Sood, A. (2015). Enhancing resilience among new nurses: Feasibility and efficacy of a pilot intervention. *Ochsner Journal, 15*(1), 38–44. Available at https://www.ncbi.nlm.nih.gov/pmc/articles/PMC4365845/

Clark, M. H., & Cundiff, N. L. (2011). Assessing the effectiveness of a college freshman seminar using propensity score adjustments. *Research in Higher Education, 52*(6), 616–639. doi:10.1007/s11162-010-9208-x

Cohen, J. (1998). A tapestry of caring: The lived experience and meaning of caring within a nursing student/faculty relationship. *Vermont Registered Nurse, 64*(3), 1–4.

Cook, D. A., Thompson, W. G., & Thomas, K. G. (2011). The Motivated Strategies for Learning Questionnaire: Score validity among medicine residents. *Medical Education, 45*(12), 1230–1240. doi:10.1111/j.1365-2923.2011.04077.x

Crookes, K., Crookes, P. A., & Walsh, K. (2013). Meaningful and engaging teaching techniques for student nurses: A literature review. *Nurse Education in Practice, 13*(4), 236–243. doi:10.1016/j.nepr.2013.04.008

Cunningham, C. J., Manier, A., Anderson, A., & Sarnosky, K. (2014). Rational versus empirical prediction of nursing student success. *Journal of Professional Nursing, 30*(6), 486–492. doi:10.1016/j.profnurs.2014.03.006

Dempsey, C., & Reilly, B. A. (2016). Nurse engagement: What are the contributing factors for success? *Online Journal of Issues in Nursing, 21*(1). Retrieved June 26, 2017, from http://www.nursingworld.org/MainMenuCategories/ANAMarketplace/ANAPeriodicals/OJIN/TableofContents/Vol-21–2016/No1-Jan-2016/Nurse-Engagement-Contributing-Factors-for-Success.html

Dewing, J. (2010). Moments of movement: Active learning and practice development. *Nurse Education in Practice, 10*(1), 22–26. doi:10.1016/j.nepr.2009.02.010

Dillon, R. S., & Stines, P. W. (1996). A phenomenological study of faculty-student caring interactions. *Journal of Nursing Education, 35*(3), 113–118. doi:10.3928/0148-4834-19960301-06

Everly, M. C. (2013). Are students' impressions of improved learning through active learning methods reflected by improved test scores? *Nursing Education Today, 33*(2), 148–151. doi:10.1016/j.nedt.2011.10.023

Friedman, B. A., & Mandel, R. G. (2009). The prediction of college student academic performance and retention: Application of expectancy and goal setting theories. *Journal of College Student Retention: Research, Theory and Practice, 11*(2), 227–246. Available at https://www.researchgate.net/publication/250145395_The_Prediction_of_College_Student_Academic_Performance_and_Retention_Application_of_Expectancy_and_Goal_Setting_Theories

Gazza, E. A., & Hunker, D. F. (2014). Facilitating student retention in online graduate nursing education programs: A review of the literature. *Nurse Education Today, 34*(7), 1125–1129. doi:10.1016/j.nedt.2014.01.010

Grant, L., & Kinman, G. (2013). The importance of emotional resilience for staff and students in the 'helping' professions: Developing an emotional curriculum. *Higher Education Academy*. Retrieved June 26, 2017, from https://www.heacademy.ac.uk/system/files/emotional_resilience_louise_grant_march_2014_0.pdf

Haas, R. E., Nugent, K. E., & Rule, R. A. (2004). The use of discriminant function analysis to predict student success on the NCLEX-RN. *Journal of Nursing Education, 43*(10), 440–446. Available at https://www.researchgate.net/publication/307882683_The_use_of_discriminant_function_analysis_to_predict_student_success_on_the_NCLEX-RN

Hart, P. L., Brannan, J. D., & De Chesnay, M. (2014). Resilience in nurses: An integrative review. *Journal of Nursing Management, 22*(6), 720–734. doi:10.1111/j.1365-2834.2012.01485.x

Herzog, S. (2014). The propensity score analytical framework: An overview and institutional research example. *New Directions for Institutional Research, No. 161.* Hoboken, NJ: Wiley Periodicals.

Hinderer, K. A., DiBartolo, M. C., & Walsh, C. M. (2014). HESI admission assessment examination scores, program progression, and NCLEX-RN success in baccalaureate nursing: An exploratory study of dependable academic indicators of success. *Journal of Professional Nursing, 30*(5), 436–442. doi:10.1016/j.profnurs.2014.01.007

Hoffman, E. M. (2014). Faculty and student relationships: Context matters. *College Teaching, 62*(1), 13–19. doi:10.1080/87567555.2013.817379

Hollinger-Smith, L. M. (2017). Reliability and validity of the Nurse Resilience Survey measures. Manuscript in preparation.

Hopkins, T. H. (2008). Early identification of at-risk nursing students: A student support model. *Journal of Nursing Education, 47*(6), 254–259. doi:10.3928/01484834-20080601-05

Johnston, J. G. (1990). The influence of English language on the ability to pass NCLEX-RN. In C. F. Waltz & O. L. Strickland (Eds.), *Measurement of Nursing Outcomes, Vol. 3: Measuring Clinical Skills and Professional Development in Education and Practice* (pp. 373–383). New York: Springer, 373–383.

Kaddoura, M. A., Flint, E. P., Van Dyke, O., Yang, Q., & Chiang, L. (2016). Academic and demographic predictors of NCLEX-RN pass rates in first- and second-degree accelerated BSN programs. *Journal of Professional Nursing, 33*(3), 229–240. doi:10.1016/j.profnurs.2016.09.005

Kan'an, A., & Osman, K. (2015). The relationship between self-directed learning skills and science achievement among Qatari students. *Creative Education, 6*(8), 790–797. Available at http://dx.doi.org/10.4236/ce.2015.68082

Kowitlawakul, Y., Brenkus, R., & Dugan, N. (2012). Predictors for success for first semester, second-degree bachelor of science in nursing students. *International Journal of Nursing Practice, 19*(Suppl. 1), 38–43. doi:10.1111/ijn.12014

Lee, Y., & Choi, J. (2011). A review of online course dropout research: Implications for practice and future research. *Educational Technology Research Development, 59*(5), 593–618. Available at https://www.learn-techlib.org/p/50902

Liljedahl, M., Bjorck, E., Kalen, S., Ponzer, S., & Laksov, K. B. (2016). To belong or not to belong: Nursing students' interactions with clinical learning environment—An observational study. *BMC Medical Education, 16*, 197–206. doi:10.1186/s12909-016-0721-2

Lucas, K. H., Testman, J. A, Hoyland, M. N., Kimble, A. M., & Euler, M. L. (2013). Correlation between active-learning coursework and student retention of core content during advanced pharmacy practice experiences. *American Journal of Pharmaceutical Education, 77*(8), 1–6. doi:10.5688/ajpe778171

Mann, J. C. (2014). A pilot study of RN-BSN completion students' preferred online classroom caring behaviors. *ABNF Journal, 25*(2), 33–39. Available at https://www.ncbi.nlm.nih.gov/pubmed/24855803

McEnroe-Petitte, D. M. (2011). Impact of faculty caring on student retention and success. *Teaching and Learning in Nursing, 6*, 80–83. doi:10.1016/j.teln.2010.12.005

McGahee, T. W., Gramling, L., & Reid, T. F. (2010). NCLEX-RN success: Are there predictors? *Southern Online Journal of Nursing Research, 10*(4). Retrieved June 26, 2017, from http://www.resourcenter.net/images/snrs/files/sojnr_articles2/vol10num04art13.html

Miller, A. S. (2007). *Students that persist: Caring relationships that make a difference in higher education.* East Lansing, MI: National Center for Research on Teacher Learning. (ERIC Document Reproduction Service No. ED497500). Available at http://www.eric.ed.gov/contentdelivery/servlet/ERICServlet?accno=ED497500

Montgomery, D. C. (2012). *Design and analysis of experiments* (8th ed.). Hoboken, NJ: Wiley.

Mooring, Q. E. (2016). Recruitment, advising, and retention programs—Challenges and solutions to the international problem of poor student retention: A narrative literature review. *Nursing Education Today, 40*, 204–208. doi:10.1016/j.nedt.2016.03.003

Nibert, A., & Young, A. (2001). A third study on predicting NCLEX success with the HESI exit exam. *Computers in Nursing, 19*(4), 172–178. doi:10.1097/01.NCN.0000336438.16918.c2

Pattison, P., Hale, J. R., & Gowens, P. (2011). Mind and soul: Connecting with students. *Journal of Legal Studies, 28*(1), 39–66. doi:10.1111/j.1744-1722.2010.01084.x

Perry, B., Boman, J., Care, W., Edwards, M., & Park, C. (2008). Why do students withdraw from online graduate nursing and health studies education? *Journal of Education Online, 5*(1), 1–17. doi:10.9743/JEO.2008.1.2

Pintrich, R. R.., & DeGroot, E. V. (1990). Motivational and self-regulated learning components of classroom academic performance. *Journal of Educational Psychology, 82*(1), 33–40. Available at http://rhartshorne.com/fall-2012/eme6507-rh/cdisturco/eme6507-eportfolio/documents/pintrich%20and%20degroodt%201990.pdf

Pintrich, P. R., Smith, D. A., Garcia, T., & McKeachie, W. J. (1993). Reliability and predictive validity of the Motivated Strategies for Learning Questionnaire (MSLQ). *Educational and Psychological Measurement, 53*(3), 801–813. doi:10.1177/0013164493053003024

Plante, K., & Asselin, M. E. (2014). Best practices for creating social presence and caring behaviors online. *Nursing Education Perspectives, 35*(4), 219–223. doi:10.5480/13-1094.1

Romeo, E. M. (2013). The predictive ability of critical thinking, nursing GPA, and SAT scores on first-time NCLEX-RN performance. *Nursing Education Perspectives, 34*(4), 248–253.

Satmetrix (2017). What is Net Promoter? Retrieved July 13, 2017 at: https://www.netpromoter.com/know/

Silvestri, L. A., Clark, M. C., & Moonie, S. A. (2013). Using logistic regression to investigate self-efficacy and the predictors for National Council Licensure Examination success for baccalaureate nursing students. *Journal of Nursing Education and Practice, 3*(6), 21–34. doi:10.5430/jnep.v3n6p21

Simmons, P. R., & Cavanaugh, S. H. (2000). Relationships among student and graduate caring ability and professional school climate. *Journal of Professional Nursing, 16*(2), 76–83.

Sitzman, K. L. (2016). What student cues prompt online instructors to offer caring interventions? *Nursing Education Perspectives, 37*(2), 61–71. doi:10.5480/14-1542

Torregosa, M. B., Ynalvez, M. A., & Morin, K. H. (2016). Perceptions matter: Faculty caring, campus racial climate and academic performance. *Journal of Advanced Nursing, 72*(4), 864–877. doi:10.1111/jan.12877

Wade, G. H., & Kasper, N. (2006). Nursing students' perceptions of instructor caring: An instrument based on Watson's Theory of Transpersonal Caring. *Journal of Nursing Education, 45*(5), 162–168. Available at https://www.researchgate.net/publication/7059333_Nursing_Students%27_Perceptions_of_Instructor_Caring_An_Instrument_Based_on_Watson%27s_Theory_of_Transpersonal_Caring

Wang, L., Tao, H., Brown, R., & Zhang, Y. (2017). Influence of social support and self-efficacy on resilience of early career registered nurses. *Western Journal of Nursing Research*. Advance online publication. doi:10.1177/0193945916685712

Willging, P., & Johnson, S. (2009). Factors that influence students' decision to dropout of online courses. *Journal of Asynchronous Learning, 13*(3), 115–127. Available at http://files.eric.ed.gov/fulltext/EJ862360.pdf

Wolkowitz, A. A., & Kelley, J. A. (2010). Academic predictors of success in a nursing program. *Journal of Nursing Education, 49*(9), 498–503. doi:10.3928/01484834-20100524-09

5

Evolving Our Culture of Care

Carla D. Sanderson, PhD, RN

CHAMBERLAIN TODAY

Today at Chamberlain, there is a pervasive demonstration of what it means to work in a culture of service excellence and care. A visit to any one of Chamberlain's 20 campuses or an online course discussion session will show evidence of what one would expect to find in the halls or online interactions of any nursing program. What stands out on Chamberlain's campuses and in its online programs are the stories you hear, the ones you have read about in these pages and countless more stories about care, and visitors commenting on a "palpable ethos."

Chamberlain has developed orientation programs aimed at equipping and encouraging all colleagues for care, as well as "Red Carpet Welcome" events for new colleagues on their first day of work. You see "Meet and Greets" for new online students and boot camps for students on writing skills and integration of anatomy and physiology knowledge. Care is shown through rapid responses by faculty to student email and phone outreach (usually within a few hours). You see faculty reaching out to students through email and phone for birthday celebrations. You see offers for special assistance and simple outreach efforts—faculty just touching base to see how their students are doing and how classes are going. You see colleagues being measured not only on what they do in their work but how they do it. You see prospective colleagues being assessed for whether they possess caring characteristics, and existing colleagues celebrated and honored for their caring behaviors. What you hear and see is *Chamberlain Care,* a laser focus on caring for students, enriched through an approach where care for self and care for colleagues come first.

The culture of care was striking to me as I was getting to know Chamberlain. Even before I was on board, I observed the faculty summit led by Ken Bain that has been previously mentioned, a highly interactive summit where faculty participated in small groups and reported new ideas for student engagement back to Dr. Bain. What I heard around small group tables was refreshing! Stories of students on faculty supporting their learning, curriculum committee members engaged in enhancements and revision, faculty reaching out to support what happens outside the classroom, and how in the face of considerable hardship, their students were being served, encouraged, and loved.

Faculty received recognition as DAISY Award recipients that day. As faculty leaders read how recipients made a particular contribution to the well-being of a student(s), I was convinced that Chamberlain *is* different. The whole picture of a student's learning needs was integrated and owned by faculty, from meeting learning outcomes to meeting personal needs for balancing work and family demands, and for belonging. What was so striking that day was who these students were. I could tell from the stories that Chamberlain enrolled a good number of students I had seldom had the opportunity to serve—students whose demands of life required full-time employment for their family, not just first-generation students breaking new ground but students for whom a college education truly seemed the impossible dream.

Most striking of all that day was the ethnic tapestry of the more than 300 faculty who filled that hotel ballroom, and the news that the Chamberlain student body made for an even more beautiful tapestry of color. Ten years prior, I had served on a PhD dissertation committee for a Latina woman who did a comprehensive literature review of health outcome improvements when the patient and nurse share ethnicity. What I saw at the faculty summit and have seen more clearly since is that Chamberlain is making a significant difference in the demographics of today's nursing workforce, which can and should result in a positive difference in the health outcomes of the demographics of the patients in their care. I signed up to be a part of *Chamberlain Care* for that.

The purpose of this final chapter on *Chamberlain Care* is fourfold: (1) *to convey our belief* that sandwiched between the crises in our higher education and health care systems is an opportunity for an ethic of care to drive solutions for both, (2) *to suggest* that educating extraordinary nurses through a culture of care is nursing education's ultimate goal, (3) *to make predictions* about the future that drive what is next for Chamberlain's research agenda and the evolution of its culture of care, and (4) *to share* tools, ideas, and activities in hopes that other institutions will collaborate with us. We are excited to partner with others toward a culture of service excellence and care in the profession of nursing—a culture that prepares students for extraordinary nursing care to persons, families, and communities.

REVISITING THE CASE FOR A CULTURE OF CARE

The leaders of Chamberlain's campuses and online programs are weaving a culture of care into the education of nurses at the baccalaureate and higher degree levels. Chamberlain gives priority to relationships with students by seeking to understand what students need and care about. Today, faculty and students are pursuing a reciprocal relationship of care as the purposes of higher education are fulfilled—to enhance intellectual exchange between faculty and students, inspiring students to learn to think and question, affecting in faculty the desire to stretch and grow to meet students where they are and take them where they need to be.

Chamberlain's seasoned nurse educators are attempting to write a new nursing education paradigm, pulling in students from the "swirl" of multiple campuses, multiple starts and stops so typical of today's higher education, and providing "academic care," modeling the concepts of care that will be required of them as graduate nurses. To fulfill the health care mandate to assess care outcomes, patients are now asked, "How well did I feel cared for?" Chamberlain believes that the capacity for the nurse to care can be affected by the care received while a nursing student.

Changing the culture at Chamberlain has been hard work. The change for Chamberlain has come in nurturing and tending to its social fabric, in communicating the expected norms and values of the *Chamberlain Care* culture, in creating a work climate where shared perceptions of care are exercised, and in fostering for Chamberlain a caring personality on every campus and in every program.

The work requires discipline, commitment, and execution of repeatable, sustainable, standardized practices and processes to support the culture of care that we envision. A keen focus on student success runs through it all, and we are "inspecting what we expect" in student success. Chamberlain serves a diverse student body where 53.8 percent of our prelicensure students have a minority background; we are developing a culture of care and a paradigm of student success with the belief that all students we admit can and should be successful. People engaging one on one with students is making a difference—an admissions counselor, a faculty member, an advisor reaching out, watching students, picking up cues, listening, coaching, mentoring, being empathetic, showing concern, offering help, demonstrating care, serving students.

A swirl of a different kind has taken place in health care—the swirl of new roles, new technologies, new financial models, new challenges, and new threats facing both hospital and community health nursing. Nurses today work in new roles and new ways in support of new aims, like the Institute for Healthcare Improvement's "triple aim," which is "improving the patient experience of care (including quality and satisfaction), improving the health of populations, and reducing the per capita cost of health care" (Seegert, 2016, pp. 18–19).

The care rendered by hospital-based nurses has shifted from episodic care to continuity of care and from provision *of* care to accountability *for* care outcomes. The risks of nursing care have broadened to include significant financial risks and liability (no funding for hospital readmissions). Rendering care in clinics, offices, retail settings, federally run health centers, and other community-based settings is equally strained due to the shifts in to whom and by whom care is provided—"brokering" equitable and accessible care through new networks and with new care providers (Davidson & Du, 2015).

Chamberlain aspires for its graduates to be extraordinary nurses, navigating change, ambiguity, and fragmentation in their work settings by working to create healthy environments of "respect, collaboration, collegiality, creativity, productivity, community and teamwork" (Chamberlain University College of Nursing Philosophy of Nursing Education). We envision our graduates replicating the caring educational culture that we are attempting to provide them, embracing a sense of meaning, wholeness, connectedness, cohesion, community, and belonging as their own paradigm of care, and becoming people of influence in their own workplaces throughout their careers.

Chamberlain Care matters as we strive to prepare people for work that matters. We all ultimately want our hard work to matter—the hard work we do as students and every day thereafter in our chosen professions. To matter is threefold: (1) to believe that we are a part of significant work, (2) to have a deep sense of personal contribution to the work, and (3) to do the work in the community with others who share our values and goals. These things come through a sense of belonging and meaningfulness engendered by the caring approach of others.

We regularly ask ourselves the question, "Is our strategic plan operationalizing our *Chamberlain Care* philosophy?" As of this writing, I am Chamberlain's newly appointed provost. In my new role, I probe our academic strategy. Are our curricula built on a foundation of care? Is every course in our general education curriculum bridging and building our BSN curriculum? Are the liberal arts inspiring students and the sciences equipping them? Is our clinical and practicum learning fully integrated through our curricula? Are we taking the best advantage of our simulation, virtual learning, and immersion experiences? Do faculty advance a culture of care through their teaching and coaching? Are our faculty caring for students in the way we would have them care for patients, families, and communities? Are faculty and leaders modeling care for colleagues to students? Is faculty scholarship building the science of care? Are our cocurricular initiatives built on a concept of care? Do our student success strategies communicate care? What are we doing to ensure that our culture of care is enlarging students' vision of themselves as agents of care? And ultimately, what ways of knowing can we use to determine if our graduates are influencing their workplaces for the good of service excellence and care?

It is our intention that engagement, collaboration, and care will be woven through-out the teaching-learning activities in our BSN, MSN, and DNP curricula. We have set an ambitious goal that our students will thrive as confident, whole individuals as they stretch to meet the rigorous requirements to complete a nursing degree. We aim for graduates to establish their identities as new, advanced practice or graduate nurses and reach their potential as contributing members and leaders of health care practice. We have work to do and much more to learn toward these ends.

NEXT STEPS IN DEVELOPING A CULTURE OF CARE

Sharpening Our Focus: An Extraordinary Nurse

Chamberlain boldly claims the goal to graduate extraordinary nurses in our purpose and vision statements, yet we recognize that the term *extraordinary* is not explicitly defined in our statements nor in the literature. A full understanding of what we mean by extraordinary is an important next step in the work of creating a culture of care in which students become extraordinary nurses. We want to improve on our model by taking an outward look to gain a clear picture of what an extraordinary nurse looks like.

In early 2017, Chamberlain's Office of Institutional Effectiveness and Research launched a study entitled *Employer and Patient Perspectives on the Characteristics, Behaviors, and Impact of Extraordinary Nurses.* Using a mixed-methods approach through focus groups and survey methods, we are exploring the perspectives of employers and patients on the characteristics, behaviors, and impact of extraordi-nary nurses. Example interview guide questions for the focus groups are found in Box 5.1. In addition, employers will be surveyed to determine how well Chamberlain graduates exemplify the extraordinary nurse. Findings from our study will expand the knowledge base of what constitutes an extraordinary nurse; better position us to align our faculty development, nursing curricula, and student success initiatives to our vision for preparing extraordinary nurses; and ultimately graduate nurses we know are valued by employers and patients alike. Our research questions are as follows:

➤ How do employers and patients describe the characteristics, behaviors, and impact of extraordinary nurses?

> How do employers rate the quality of Chamberlain graduates relative to identified characteristics and behaviors of extraordinary nurses?

> What recommendations do employers and patients offer Chamberlain on how to best prepare extraordinary nurses?

The research findings will advance Chamberlain's aspiration to prepare extraordinary nurses who embrace the caring imperative of practice through meaningful relationships with others. Care is a relationship. "The mandate is clear for a nursing practice that is based on the intention to know persons more fully as human beings, transcending the notion of persons as objects of care. The nurse is challenged to know persons as whole using every possible creative, imaginative, and innovative way to appreciate and celebrate their intentions. Nurses need to return to an overriding imperative of practice to know persons more fully as whole in order to maintain and sustain their humanness" (Locsin & Purnell, 2015, p. 52).

We desire to instill in graduates an appreciation for the rich and diverse opportunities that will be afforded them in relationship with those in their care. Braced with scientific knowledge and the resources for critical examination of health and illness, Chamberlain is working to equip its graduates for extraordinary care in relationships that help patients and their families encounter life's most intimate moments, both those that are difficult and those most meaningful.

Extraordinary nursing care is a philosophic enterprise—a thinking and searching activity. We want to help students find their voice and become nurses who will commit themselves to take a bold stance for what is right and good, and against what is wrong. Extraordinary nurses can be empowered through their roles as primary patient advocates to speak up in the face of sweeping changes in health care delivery. Extraordinary nurses will get involved in the profession's organizations and work to influence policies and legislation that impact health care and affect the lives of patients. Extraordinary nurses embody a commitment, not only to think and act wisely in the administration of therapeutic nursing interventions but also to think and act in accordance with the beliefs

BOX 5.1

Extraordinary Nurse Study: Example Interview Guide Questions for Focus Groups

1. What makes a nurse extraordinary?
2. When you think of a nurse giving extraordinary care, what does that look like?
3. How does the extraordinary nurse approach his or her nursing care differently than the typical nurse?
4. Describe how the extraordinary nurse interacts with patients, families, and coworkers differently than the typical nurse.
5. How are others (patients, families, coworkers, employers) impacted by the care of an extraordinary nurse?
6. What more can you say to describe an extraordinary nurse?
7. How might Chamberlain best ensure the preparation of future extraordinary nurses?

and values of the profession. We seek to graduate extraordinary nurses who are ready to make a profound impact through exercising *Chamberlain Care.*

Sharpening Our Focus: Extraordinary Faculty

In Chapter 3, we described a culture of care for faculty. Chamberlain is working its vision for developing extraordinary faculty who learn about themselves as teachers in order to develop the competencies needed for transformative teaching-learning relationships with students. We aim for a relationship with faculty based on trust, respect, and a shared sense of meaning and purpose, one that recognizes faculty for giving their best effort to advance the *Chamberlain Care* core values. An extraordinary faculty member both receives and provides coaching and mentoring in community with fellow faculty. And from there, extraordinary faculty engage in lively interactions with students, accompanying them on their journey of learning, caring for and about them, bringing learning into their lives, understanding how they learn, and working to meet their individual learning needs. Extraordinary faculty are the greatest influencers of student success, demonstrating integrity and professionalism in all manners of behavior, participating in active learning with them, and modeling for them the values of service excellence and care.

Essentials in Developing Extraordinary Faculty: Lessons Learned

The following aspirations for faculty will help shape our planning going forward, as will the lessons that we have learned thus far. What follows is a list of essentials that we have identified along the way in our goal of preparing extraordinary faculty:

> *Hiring:* Hiring for *Chamberlain Care*'s mission and values is the first and most important step in our goal of developing extraordinary faculty. We search for faculty who have the potential to emulate *Chamberlain Care* in their interactions with colleagues, students, and external partners. Yet more work is needed to refine the selection process for hiring *Chamberlain Care* faculty. We have learned that service excellence and care in hiring means taking the time to hire, orient, and develop faculty well. We have also learned that service excellence and care also mean making tough decisions to address mistakes in hiring when they occur.

> *Work–Life Balance:* In an environment where care for self is the starting point in establishing a culture of care, genuine attention must be given to a working environment that promotes a healthy work–life balance. The human resources team plays an integral part in ensuring that we live up to what we value. Recently, the team did a comprehensive study of benefits and implemented a flex-work arrangement in response to faculty and staff needs and desires. It is challenging but imperative for a growing institution to keep a close eye on new and emerging concepts in competitive benefits for colleagues.

> *An Ethnically Diverse Faculty:* Advocacy for an ethnically diverse faculty that mirrors our ethnically diverse student body is an essential part of *Chamberlain Care.* We will continue our commitment to faculty diversity, finding ways to bring graduates back to teach on our campuses and in our programs.

> *Part-Time Faculty Are Significant Faculty, Too:* The quality of interactions with students for visiting faculty is as critical as full-time faculty interactions, especially in the clinical environment and online. Although we have a strong new faculty orientation program for visiting professors, and engagement scores that exceed benchmark scores for the best companies in the world (even higher than our full-time faculty), we need to do a better job of building community with them and developing them in the Chamberlain culture of care. There are models of engagement with visiting professors throughout Chamberlain, such as face-to-face visiting professor summits designed to reinforce the concepts of *Chamberlain Care.* These models need to be standardized and offered on all campuses and in all online programs.

> *Be on Message:* It is not enough to send an email or memorandum to faculty when promoting a new *Chamberlain Care* teaching-learning strategy or student engagement tips. Faculty need to question, test, critique, and probe for deep understanding before they will adopt change. And this is good news! Messaging efforts need to be planned well, giving time for dialogue and experimentation. We have learned that messaging needs to be sustained through online and face-to-face dialogue, workshops, and reinforcement initiatives. We have seen that once faculty *own Chamberlain Care* as their own philosophy and attitude toward teaching and learning, the culture of care becomes palpable and the model advances.

> *Monitoring Toil:* Becoming excellent is hard work, *especially* for faculty. We must continue to acknowledge the hard work that is taking place—the trial-and-error testing that comes with becoming an excellent teacher. We made a mistake in the implementation of a student success strategy, a mistake that touched every campus and affected student success metrics on multiple cohorts of students. The mistake took a toll on morale. We responded with transparency, owning the mistake and calling the faculty to work their way through it. We learned the necessity of meticulous change management oversight.

> *Tending the Social Fabric:* Care for colleagues is ever important during a time of significant change. Our president visits each campus and spends time with all online colleagues at least once a year, and usually more often in what she calls "The Roadshow." Although the purpose is to communicate her vision, give college-wide updates, and inform colleagues about important changes, we have learned that the real value-added benefit is bringing people together, making connections, promoting community, and increasing morale. We have learned that the culture of care to which we aspire gets stronger with each social encounter and community-building activity we offer.

Sharpening Our Focus: Extraordinary Students

In Chapter 4, we described a culture of care for students that is based on the "fundamental belief in the college's responsibility and ability to achieve superior student outcomes for a diverse population of students...through initiatives that lead to...extraordinary care, strong support for each student's learning experience, motivating actions instead of demotivating actions and encouragement instead of discouragement in the face of challenges" (Chamberlain University College of Nursing Philosophy of Nursing Education). Accordingly, Chamberlain is working its vision for developing extraordinary students to be self-determined, accountable, confident, and courageous. An extraordinary student would be one who seeks out knowledge and learns to apply it in new ways to develop the critical thinking and problem solving skills required of the professional nurse. The extraordinary student accepts his or her program's invitation to engage, to get involved, interact with faculty, and build community with fellow students. Higher education is a relationship. The extraordinary student would find *belonging* in relationships at Chamberlain, and Chamberlain would offer belonging to students for a lifetime by striving to meet ongoing learning needs.

Essentials in Developing Extraordinary Students: Lessons Learned

With the following aspirations for students as our goal, we continue to explore and study what it will take to reach them. What follows is another list of essentials, which are identified as being key in achieving our goal of preparing extraordinary students:

> ▸ **Prioritizing Student Success:** Terrell Strayhorn, the Ohio State student success scholar and author of *College Students' Sense of Belonging* (2012), recently tweeted, "Access without success is useless." We work hard to strike the right balance between access and success. We know that *Chamberlain Care* does not mean that every prelicensure applicant who wants to be a nurse should be admitted, but we are deeply committed to discovering new ways for determining student potential for success. For instance, knowing that the standardized ACT entrance exam is not normed on the majority of students we admit, we have looked for different meaningful measures. As discussed in Chapter 4, we embarked on extensive studies to determine better metrics to predict student success coming in and stronger academic and nonacademic assessments to predict the likelihood of successful student outcomes in the end. Yet we have much more to learn— our licensure and certification pass rates do not meet the bar that we have set for ourselves. We will address next steps in determining student success in a discussion of our research agenda to follow.

> ▸ **Addressing Student Swirl:** A very strong majority of our students transfer credits from institutions they attended before Chamberlain. Chamberlain students are typical of the student swirl described earlier in this chapter. *Academically Adrift: Limited Learning on College Campuses* (Arum and Roksa, 2010) provides discourse on low average learning among today's college students. Arum and Roksa's study of 2,300 students suggests that 45 percent of students experience no learning gains in skills such as critical thinking and complex reasoning (p. 41). We cannot make assumptions about the credits students have been awarded in the prerequisite courses they bring to Chamberlain, and we are looking to educational technology for new ways to ensure mastery of essential content in nursing education.

> ▸ **Meeting Students Where They Are: Academic Planning:** On average, Chamberlain students are older, work full time, and have significant family responsibilities. Many come to us highly stressed by prior attempts to be enrolled

in a nursing program. We have learned to pay attention to both academic and work–life factors, working within the reality of the students' situations and not trying to work around them. To address the academic demands, we have learned to maintain as much flexibility as possible in our curriculum mapping to accommodate students as needed. We are eager to explore what new educational technologies offer us in providing targeted individualized learning.

> *Meeting Students Where They Are: Intrusive Advising:* To address the work–life demands, we depend on student services advisors to demonstrate *Chamberlain Care* to students one on one through careful planning and advising; we borrowed the phrase "intrusive advising" to describe the action-oriented approach that these advisors take to learn what is causing difficulty for a student and problem solve the difficulties with them (Earl, 1988). Student services advisors think through creative options for scheduling courses and employment, solving for immediate financial needs and coaching through interpersonal challenges with faculty and fellow students—in essence, providing the needed glue and cohesion that was mentioned previously in this chapter. We are proactive with students in helping them strategize repayment of their education debt, but the demands of student employment continue to be a significant challenge. We would like to formalize alliances with employers of nursing to provide meaningful, complementary work options more available to those students who need to work.

> *Meeting Students Where They Are: Interventional Care:* In Chapter 4, our new Chamberlain Early Assessment Program (CEAP) was discussed. We have learned to pay attention to nonacademic matters such as scores indicating challenges with critical thinking, test taking, resiliency, the English language, family demands, and emotional stress. Our work in interventional research to find ways to address these challenges, thereby offering "interventional care," is just beginning.

> *Navigating Across Cultures:* Chamberlain has given emphasis to an attitude of cultural humility, "an active process, an ongoing way of being in the world and being in relationships with others and self" (Miller, 2009, p. 92), in the Chamberlain University College of Nursing Philosophy of Nursing Education. We are privileged to serve students from many different cultures and know our student body will become increasingly diverse in the years ahead. We are committed to learning how to better navigate the disparities that exist between the cultures represented in our classrooms and online. For instance, Chamberlain's online academicians are finding ways to offer a one-to-one coach or "navigator" for postlicensure students identified as higher-risk on admission by virtue of English language understanding (and also by virtue of a lower GPA or lack of clinical work experience). We have audited our curriculum for cultural biases and are hosting weekly language and culture immersion options on campuses. Interventional care to include bridging cultural disparity is an area of focus for us.

> *Funding Retention:* To be faithful to the values of *Chamberlain Care,* we are committed to retaining every student we admit who can demonstrate achievement of learning outcomes. We lose students most often because the demands of their work and family responsibilities do not afford them adequate time for study. But we do not expect or easily accept losing students. We have learned that a

mind-set of working hard for academic success in every student leads to improved retention. So we find a way to fund cocurricular initiatives, such as having a Center for Academic Success on every campus and writing boot camps for graduate students. Funding for the next phase of the CEAP is an emerging priority, helping students address and even overcome nonacademic barriers to their progression in nursing education.

> *Watching for Cues:* Terrell Strayhorn, speaking at the 2017 Annual Meeting of the Higher Learning Commission, said "A sigh is the universal sound of distress." We have learned to watch students for cues, reading tone, and listening for indications of stress—like sighing, watching for cynicism, anger, and other signs of nonproductive behavior—and anticipating student need. We know that teaching students *Chamberlain Care*'s care for self while in school will contribute to their success as a student and to their ongoing development and advancement in the nursing profession. We want to improve in this area, focusing students on becoming whole persons through care-for-self experiential learning activities and professional development in our courses and across our curricula.

> *Be on Message:* In *The End of College: Creating the Future of Learning and the University of Everywhere,* Kevin Carey states that "clarity of purpose is the single most important quality a program can have" (2015, p. 247). We have seen students latch on to *Chamberlain Care.* We work hard to message that we are a college with one priority—graduating extraordinary health care professionals. We strive to send a concise and coherent sense of who Chamberlain is in the way we promote ourselves, specifically what we are trying to accomplish on behalf of students— care, extraordinary graduates, nurses equipped to transform health care worldwide. We are now facing the challenge of extending that message as we transition to Chamberlain University.

> *Student Ambassadors for Chamberlain Care:* We described the *Net Promoter Score* (NPS) tool in Chapter 4, which is the metric we use to determine students' likelihood of recommending us to others. We hear stories from students that *Chamberlain Care* is important to them, but we have not been able to increase our prelicensure student NPS despite our messaging and care interventions, whereas NPS scores among postlicensure students are very high. We recognize that when an individual is experiencing the level of stress and challenge that prelicensure nursing education creates, his or her sensitivities are more inwardly than outwardly focused. Postlicensure students are working nurses who are better able to balance work, school, and life. Is that it? We know that many of our students are at Chamberlain because a graduate told them about us. Is it that the NPS would be higher among our graduates? We want to learn more about true student and graduate perception of *Chamberlain Care.*

> *Belonging Matters:* As mentioned previously, people want to belong to something and someone, some community. If we had to choose one lesson learned on which to build our next steps, the lesson that belonging matters to students might be it. Habits of heart and mind formed in community nurture a life of integrity and significance. Belonging in community comes when students find a mentor (faculty, advisor, coach) whose life demonstrates something extraordinary that they want

to emulate and when they find friends to bear them up and hold them accountable in meeting their goals. Many students have natural strengths that lead them to find belonging, but some do not. We want to find ways to foster belonging at Chamberlain for those students, like dividing online students into smaller pods of five to six students for threaded discussions, where faculty and fellow students can interact more intimately in small groups.

We trust that the essentials for developing faculty and students that have been identified and the lessons learned through our experiences with them are generalizable and replicable for our readers.

We readily admit that *Chamberlain Care* has not solved all problems and that operational issues can threaten to overwhelm the culture we are trying to create. We admit that the work we are doing is very hard work, and that sometimes we get tired. But on a day-to-day basis, we are experiencing a culture with an atmosphere of cooperation, trust, and collegiality whereby we address and solve problems together, most often enthusiastically and with a positive attitude. At the end of the day, there is a sense of commitment to students, to the college, and to one another to work out our shared problems and prevail in our shared mission. People believe that being excellent and extraordinary is hard work but a worthy goal to which they want to contribute, and they enjoy doing the work of *Chamberlain Care* in community with other people who believe the same thing.

A Call for Collaboration in Integrating Care Cultures in Nursing Education and Practice

Predictions About Future Needs of Students, Faculty, and Employers

In 2016, the *Chronicle of Higher Education* published Jeffrey Selingo's work, *2026—The Decade Ahead: The Seismic Shifts Transforming the Future of Higher Education* (Selingo 2016b). Selingo forecasts the shifting demographics and declining socioeconomic factors that will affect college enrollments and our learners of the future. He outlines the "existential questions about the future of the faculty and a dizzying array of technology options for teaching learning" (p. 40). To read his work with a hopeful eye, we can see great opportunity, challenging yet powerful—the ethnically diverse student body that is needed to provide optimum care for our ethnically diverse society, the eager student hungry for the vocational opportunity to increase the well-being of his or her family; and bifurcated faculty, those faculty hired for teaching, and those hired for scholarship, where teaching faculty are paired up with preceptors, teaching assistants, and instructional designers (Chamberlain is doing some of this now); and added to eager students and teaching faculty will be amazing technological advances with teaching-learning resources adapted to individual student learning styles and learning needs.

Kevin Carey, in *The End of College* (2015), describes the future technological landscape as one where educational computer engineers will work with faculty to assess and adapt the pace and progress of student learning through "customization and personalization, the product of artificial intelligence, the ability to create digital learning environments where the educational design changes based on the learner himself ... if

I arrive in a course with a serious deficit in chemistry knowledge, the computer figures that out and changes the lectures I watch and problems I solve accordingly, or puts me in a discussion group with other students who can help me learn...instead of just making me 'Wrong,' it reroutes the learning process like a car GPS that calculates a new route to your destination after you've made a wrong turn" (p. 103).

Jeffrey Selingo, in *Life After College* (2016a), focuses on the soft skills that higher education will need to attend to in the future—curiosity, sharing, negotiating, contextual thinking, and humility. Selingo contends that with the world of work changing faster than ever due to technological advances (what he calls the *gig economy*), significant change will need to occur to equip students with the soft skills to be successful navigating the ambiguity that rapid change brings. We can be confident that nursing will not disappear because of technological advances and artificial intelligence, but we can be just as confident that automation in the classroom and workplace will change what students need to know and are able to do.

As a final thought about what we can expect to see in the future, employers cannot afford the time and expense of hiring people who are not adaptable to new workplace realities. Higher education must address the mismatch between what students bring to their jobs and what employers expect. As Chamberlain has begun to see, employers will increasingly find their own way to educate their employees through alliances and partnerships.

Planning for the Future: Evolving a Culture of Care

The Institute of Medicine's 2011 *Future of Nursing* report called us to "embrace technology, foster partnerships, encourage collaboration across disciplines and settings, ensure continuity of care and promote nurse-led/nurse managed health care" (p. 402). With that in mind, the following ideas are guides in the ongoing evolution of a culture of service excellence and care:

▸ ***Transformational Teaching-Learning:*** Prioritizing academic technologies to address student success through implementing the "GPS" adaptive learning approach mentioned previously, connecting to the best-in-field master teachers via videoconferencing, scaling learning remotely by providing outstanding clinical learning via robotic telepresence (which is different from the virtual avatar learning available today), and linking students in online courses to a whole new world of educational opportunities via new collaboration tools—not only can we think one to one and one to many, but we can now think many to many (Cortez, 2017).

▸ ***Partnerships:*** Building on existing partnerships for clinical learning, build alliances and coalitions within health care institutions that assign responsibility to each for what they do best—in our case, meeting educational learning needs across the partnership as opposed to each partner offering some level of education on its own.

▸ ***Interprofessional Collaboration:*** Fostering interprofessional collaboration through simulation centers where students from the health professions explore a culture of care in complex clinical and community situations, building the scholarship of interprofessional care, starting with the professions of nursing, medicine, and public health.

> **Rural Workforce Needs:** Transforming our metropolitan area prelicensure education model to meet needs for more nurses in rural, underserved areas in the nation, facilitating continuity of care in places that may be difficult to access.

> **Student Success:** Fully integrating propensity modeling as the essence of our student success model, both at prelicensure and postlicensure levels, using the model to further refine and build a more robust and effective student support and intervention system.

> **The Voice of a Leader:** Weaving professionalism, accountability and responsibility more strategically into *Chamberlain Care,* teaching new leadership essentials such as thriving in chaos and navigating the ambiguity of managed care, stretching students in the activities of enlarging, navigating, connecting, reproducing, and multiplying, emboldening them to speak up for what is right and good in service to patients, families, and communities.

> **Information Science:** Taking the next step in moving nursing and health care research to the bedside by preparing information scientists who can work with data to predict and provide individualized care for patients (i.e., modeling clinical data to predict and prevent individual patient risk and using data to raise nursing care standards).

> **Instilling Lifelong Belonging:** Building Chamberlain's space for lifelong learning where Chamberlain's graduates enter, leave, and reenter according to new workplace learning requirements and needs, staying connected to the *Chamberlain Care* culture to earn new knowledge and skills, and receiving "stackable credentials" across the span of their professional career.

Planning for the Future: An Agenda for Research

Going forward, Chamberlain will continue to pursue its questions and seek to solve its challenges through the use of data and evidence as an important means of understanding. Ideas for the next steps in a culture of care research agenda include the following actions:

> Develop rigorous research designs using the propensity modeling methodology in which the objective is to elucidate cause–effect student success relationships.

> Study the effectiveness of *Chamberlain Care* in promoting student success and desired student learning outcomes.

> Explore students' perceptions, attitudes, and beliefs about a culture of care and their experiences with *Chamberlain Care* in supporting a caring academic culture.

> Explore clinical and community partners' perceptions, attitudes, and beliefs about *Chamberlain Care*'s ability to foster a caring workplace culture.

> Develop and test a *Chamberlain Care* curriculum for community/clinical partners.

> Define care for self and care for colleagues, identifying the impact they both have on faculty outcome exemplars and faculty retention.

> Examine interprofessional collaboration between nursing, medicine, and public health and its impact on student readiness to meet local community needs.

> ➤ Further explore the effect principles of *Master Instruction* have on student learning outcomes.

> ➤ Identify what type(s) of "meaningful recognition" has the most impact on faculty engagement, achievement, and retention.

> ➤ Engage in other research activities to strengthen research findings in the area of student success and beyond:

>> ➤ Implement studies with methodologies that generate findings beyond description and association to findings that establish causative and predictive factors for student success.

>> ➤ Standardize definitions and measures of retention and persistence so that comparisons of results across programs and institutions can be more accurately made.

>> ➤ Obtain stronger evidence to support discernment and application of best educational practices.

>> ➤ Implement psychometric testing to develop more reliable and valid measurement tools.

>> ➤ Use more direct measures of student learning outcomes as opposed to reliance on indirect measures (i.e., course grades, student satisfaction).

>> ➤ Implement qualitative studies that move beyond simple description and more firmly establish a theoretical basis for student success quality improvement and /or evaluation studies.

Looking for Partners: Tools and Activities to Promote a Culture of Care

Advancing the culture of service excellence and care described here requires the sharing of ideas, tools, and activities with those seeking to integrate a care model into their educational program or workplace setting. Culture-shaping work requires deep conviction and careful deliberation.

We commend the American Association of Critical-Care Nurses (AACN) Healthy Work Environments Toolkit found at https://www.aacn.org/nursing-excellence/healthy-work-environments/hwe-resources for review and consideration. This guide is based on AACN Standards for Establishing and Sustaining Healthy Work Environments: A Journey to Excellence, which emphasizes standards in skilled communication, true collaboration, effective decision making, appropriate staffing, meaningful recognition, and authentic leadership as "ingredients for success." The toolkit is an evidence-based manual developed by Alissa Samoya, DNP, RN, CPN, to be used as a complementary guide for leaders striving to improve the work environment of nurses. It has readings, assessments, discussion guides, facilitation tools, and action plans to complete. We resonate with the AACN's very comprehensive approach to transforming a culture.

To give a specific focus to a culture of care, we recommend that leaders and teams engage in discussion around culture-shaping topics as follows:

> ➤ *Culture*

>> ➤ What do you assume about the way your organization is? About the way it should be?

> ➤ What does your organization make possible? What does it make difficult, if not impossible?
> ➤ What are the core values of your organization?
> ➤ What words describe your culture?
> ➤ What are the traits of your culture?
> ➤ Do the words and traits that you have identified complement the core values of your organization?
> ➤ What words do you wish described about your culture?

> ➤ *Community Members (Students/Faculty/Colleagues/Employees)*
>   > ➤ What performance metrics describe your community members?
>   > ➤ Do they promote or recommend their community to their friends and family?
>   > ➤ Are your members engaged?
>   > ➤ Do they believe that they have work that matters? Make a unique and individual contribution to that work? Have a community of colleagues to enjoy the work with?
>   > ➤ How are your community members recognized for excellence?

> ➤ *An Extraordinary Nurse*
>   > ➤ Identify three extraordinary nurses you know, each working in a different health care setting, and identify his or her five most extraordinary characteristics.
>   > ➤ Which of these characteristics are learned versus naturally acquired?
>   > ➤ Using this information, write a definition of extraordinary nurse.
>   > ➤ Draft a plan for the development of an extraordinary nurse.

A CALL FOR LEADERSHIP

Leaders give purposeful definition to vision, core values, mission, and strategy, and in doing so they shape the future of the organizations they lead. Before leaders know what the future will be, they must first fully understand what the present is like. The leader's role begins with defining reality, and acknowledging and owning the set of circumstances, challenges, and risks inherent in the work that lies ahead. Knowing and embracing the reality of where you are is essential to leading forward toward where you want to be.

The reality for Chamberlain was the plight of students who came to us with the "dream of a career and a better life for themselves and families" against the low odds of realizing their dreams given the challenges in traditional nursing education. We wanted Chamberlain to be a place where they could be successful.

Organizational culture, in the context of this writing, is the "lens through which all college operations, processes, practices, behaviors and interactions are viewed and assessed" (Chamberlain University College of Nursing Philosophy of Nursing Education). We are working to advance a culture at our organization by cultivating the ideals of care and holding ourselves accountable for the execution of the practices of care. The concept of cultivation is the forward-focused activity inherent in culture making—creating the most fertile conditions possible to grow your organization to the place you want to be. Cultivating culture is about surviving and thriving, and about culture making and culture keeping.

Jim Collins, in his book *Good to Great* (2001), describes three tiers in the process of getting to the place you want to be—"disciplined people...disciplined thought...disciplined action" (p. 142). Sometimes it seems like there is not enough discipline to be found to get us where we want to be. "The change will take too long," we tell ourselves; "I don't have the right people to make this happen," we often worry.

Leaders think comprehensively and plan incrementally when involved in culture-shaping work. It has been said that we sometimes overestimate what can be accomplished in one year while underestimating what can be accomplished in five years. The cultivation work is never ending, but the goal is ever fresh and compelling. "At Chamberlain, we are inspired, humbled, and challenged by the opportunity and responsibility we have to help our students achieve their goals and reach their dreams, and to graduate extraordinary nurses who will transform health care worldwide" (Groenwald, 2017).

References

American Association of Critical-Care Nurses (AACN) Healthy Work Environments Toolkit found at https://www.aacn.org/nursing-excellence/health-work-environments/hwe-resources

Arum, R., & Roksa, J. (2010). *Academically adrift: Limited learning on college campuses.* Chicago: University of Chicago Press.

Carey, K. (2015). *The end of college: Creating the future of learning and the University of Everywhere.* New York: Riverhead Books.

Chamberlain University College of Nursing Philosophy of Nursing Education, Chamberlain College of Nursing Academic Catalog. http://chamberlain.edu/docs/default-source/academics-admissions/catalog.pdf?sfvrsn=288, pages 18–19.

Collins, J. (2001). *Good to great.* New York: HarperCollins.

Cortez, M. B. (2017). *3 innovations borne out of virtual classrooms expand higher education's reach: Efforts to increase online collaboration spark cutting edge solutions.* Retrieved June 26, 2017, from https://www-edtechmag-azine-com.cdn.ampproject.org/c/www.edtechmagazine.com/higher/article/2017/03/3-innovations-borne-out-virtual-classrooms-expand-higher-education-s-reach?amp

Davidson, P. M., & Du, H. (2015). Nurses do not have proprietary rights on caring: But we do on clinical practice models. *Journal of Nursing Management, 23*(4), 409–410. doi:10.1111/jonm.12299

Earl, W. R. (1988). Intrusive advising of freshmen in academic difficulty. *NACADA Journal, 8*(2), 27–33. doi:10.12930/0271–9517–8.2.27

Groenwald, S. (2017). Personal correspondence.

Institute of Medicine. (2011). *The future of nursing: Leading change, advancing health.* Washington, DC: National Academies Press.

Locsin, R., & Purnell, M. (2015). Advancing the theory of technological competency as caring in nursing: The universal technological domain. *International Journal for Human Care, 19*(2), 50–54.

Miller, S. (2009). Cultural humility is the first step to becoming global care providers. *Journal of Obstetric, Gynecologic, and Neonatal Nursing, 38*(1), 92–93.

Seegert, L. (2016). New models transform care and nursing roles: More opportunities for NPs to be full partners. *AJN Reports, 116*(3), 18–19. doi:10.1097/01.NAJ.0000481270.84439.ef

Selingo, J. (2016a). *Life after college.* New York: HarperCollins.

Selingo, J. (2016b). 2026—The decade ahead: The seismic shifts transforming the future of higher education. *Chronicle of Higher Education.* Retrieved June 26, 2017, from http://chronicle.texterity.com/chronicle/2026_report?pg=1#pg1

Strayhorn, T. (2012). *College students' sense of belonging.* New York: Routledge.

Master Instruction
Classroom Observation

COLLEGE *of* NURSING

National Management Office | 3005 Highland Parkway, Downers Grove, IL 60515 | 888.556.8226 | chamberlain.edu
Please visit **chamberlain.edu/locations** for location specific address, phone and fax information.

MASTER INSTRUCTION
CLASSROOM OBSERVATION

Master Instruction Classroom Observation is designed to advance the practice of *Master Instruction* through self-reflection and peer observation of campus-based and online faculty. Integral to *Master Instruction* is creating a positive, participatory learning environment through deliberate use of evidence-based strategies to foster deep student learning. Self and dialogic reflection expands perspectives to confront and resolve actual and desired teaching practices and facilitate successful student learning outcomes. The descriptors found in this survey are characteristics of *Master Instruction* and not specific tasks. Through self-reflection, the individual faculty member must interpret the criterion in the way that best meets the learning objective, content to be delivered and learning environment setting. Prior to the observation, the designated observer will review the self-reflection of the faculty member and then observe the faculty-student interaction and provide detailed feedback of the observation to promote professional development.

Directions

Faculty are required to validate completion of the *Master Instruction* Classroom Observation process twice per fiscal year. A Likert scale is used to record observation responses of each characteristic of *Master Instruction* to guide professional development only, it is not intended to serve as a performance evaluation. The observer must provide specific examples for each characteristic of *Master Instruction* to guide dialogue to advance the practice of *Master Instruction*. Following the observation, the observer will share their insights from the review with the faculty member in a private meeting. The purpose of this meeting is to expand perspectives through dialogic reflection to transform teaching practices. The faculty member will also reflect upon and rate his/her practice of *Master Instruction* to guide professional development.

Please fill out the following fields:

Instructor Name: _____

Course (ex: NR-101): _____

Instructor DSI Number (ex: DI 2345678): _____

Instructor Email: _____

Observer Name: _____

Observer Title: _____

Date of Observation (MM/DD/YYYY): _____

COLLEGE *of* NURSING

National Management Office | 3005 Highland Parkway, Downers Grove, IL 60515 | 888.556.8226 | chamberlain.edu

Please visit **chamberlain.edu/locations** for location specific address, phone and fax information.

MASTER INSTRUCTION
CLASSROOM OBSERVATION

Please select the session from the list below:

☐ July 2016	☐ May 2017	☐ March 2018
☐ September 2016	☐ July 2017	☐ May 2018
☐ November 2016	☐ September 2017	☐ July 2018
☐ January 2017	☐ November 2017	☐ September 2018
☐ March 2017	☐ January 2018	☐ November 2018

Was this your first or second observation?   ☐ First   ☐ Second

Please select your location from the list below:

☐ Addison	☐ Indianapolis	☐ St. Louis
☐ Arlington	☐ Irving	☐ Tinley Park
☐ Atlanta	☐ Jacksonville	☐ Troy
☐ Charlotte	☐ Las Vegas	☐ Pre-Licensure Online
☐ Chicago	☐ Miramar	☐ RN to BSN Online
☐ Cleveland	☐ North Brunswick	☐ MSN Online (Non-FNP)
☐ Columbus Onsite	☐ Pearland	☐ FNP Online
☐ Columbus Online (Pre-Licensure)	☐ Phoenix	☐ DNP Online
☐ Houston	☐ Sacramento	

COLLEGE *of* NURSING

National Management Office | 3005 Highland Parkway, Downers Grove, IL 60515 | 888.556.8226 | chamberlain.edu
Please visit **chamberlain.edu/locations** for location specific address, phone and fax information.

MASTER INSTRUCTION
CLASSROOM OBSERVATION

For the next 6 questions, please use the following scale:

1 – Does not fully meet expected results: Results in important areas are not being met. Significant development and improvement in results and/or behaviors are necessary.

2 – Still developing in achieving results: Achieves results in some areas and requires development in other areas. May need more consistency at times in achieving results. Some additional development and improvement in results and/or behaviors is necessary in targeted areas.

3 – Fully effective/achieves expected results: Solid performance. Fulfills all expected results and behaviors. Generates results above those expected of the position in some areas.

4 – Exceeds expected results: Outstanding performance almost without exception. Consistently demonstrates exceptional results and behaviors above what is expected of the position.

Content Management	1 – Does Not Fully Meet Expected Results	2 – Still Developing in Achieving Results	3 – Fully Effective/Achieves Expected Results	4 – Exceeds Expected Results
• Relevant content, appropriately rigorous and applied to real life concepts • Explains how assignments and evaluation methods support course objectives • Is prepared, current, credible, knowledgeable	☐	☐	☐	☐

Comments (include specific details):

_____

_____

_____

_____

0717pflcp

COLLEGE *of* NURSING

National Management Office | 3005 Highland Parkway, Downers Grove, IL 60515 | 888.556.8226 | chamberlain.edu
Please visit **chamberlain.edu/locations** for location specific address, phone and fax information.

MASTER INSTRUCTION
CLASSROOM OBSERVATION

Active Learning	1 – Does Not Fully Meet Expected Results	2 – Still Developing in Achieving Results	3 – Fully Effective/Achieves Expected Results	4 – Exceeds Expected Results
• Engages students and holds their attention • Challenges them to rethink their assumptions • Uses multiple methods to promote learning	☐	☐	☐	☐

Comments (include specific details):

_____

_____

_____

_____

Relevance	1 – Does Not Fully Meet Expected Results	2 – Still Developing in Achieving Results	3 – Fully Effective/Achieves Expected Results	4 – Exceeds Expected Results
• Application of materials • Moves deliberately through Bloom's taxonomy • Guides the use of scholarly work from the profession • Uses evaluation methods that promote lifelong learning	☐	☐	☐	☐

Comments (include specific details):

_____

_____

_____

_____

COLLEGE *of* NURSING

National Management Office | 3005 Highland Parkway, Downers Grove, IL 60515 | 888.556.8226 | chamberlain.edu
Please visit **chamberlain.edu/locations** for location specific address, phone and fax information.

MASTER INSTRUCTION
CLASSROOM OBSERVATION

Facilitation	1 – Does Not Fully Meet Expected Results	2 – Still Developing in Achieving Results	3 – Fully Effective/Achieves Expected Results	4 – Exceeds Expected Results
• Uses a respond-extend-probe discussion model • Allows students opportunities for trial/error feedback in advance of summative judgment of their work	☐	☐	☐	☐

Comments (include specific details):

_____

_____

_____

_____

Integration	1 – Does Not Fully Meet Expected Results	2 – Still Developing in Achieving Results	3 – Fully Effective/Achieves Expected Results	4 – Exceeds Expected Results
• Promotes learning outside the classroom • Promotes curiosity with challenging questions, frequent feedback	☐	☐	☐	☐

Comments (include specific details):

_____

_____

_____

_____

COLLEGE *of* NURSING

National Management Office | 3005 Highland Parkway, Downers Grove, IL 60515 | 888.556.8226 | chamberlain.edu
Please visit **chamberlain.edu/locations** for location specific address, phone and fax information.

MASTER INSTRUCTION
CLASSROOM OBSERVATION

Classroom Environment	1 – Does Not Fully Meet Expected Results	2 – Still Developing in Achieving Results	3 – Fully Effective/Achieves Expected Results	4 – Exceeds Expected Results
• Reinforces the learning agreement • Fosters a learning spirit; promotes civility and professionalism	☐	☐	☐	☐

Comments (include specific details):

_____

_____

_____

_____

What was done especially well during the observation?

_____

_____

_____

_____

_____

What are opportunities to transform teaching practices?

_____

_____

_____

_____

_____

Please provide an overall rating of the instructor's practice of *Master Instruction*:

☐ 1 – Does not fully meet expected results   ☐ 3 – Fully effective/achieves expected results

☐ 2 – Still developing in achieving results   ☐ 4 – Exceeds expected results

P-XXXX
Master Instruction Classroom Observation_12-XXXXXX_FRM

Date 07/07/17	Printed At 100%	Agency PF
Time 5:00 PM	Round 1	

Job info

Element	Form		Pages	6 pg
Live	8.5" x 11"		Folded Size	
Trim	8.5" x 11"		VDP	☐
Bleed	.125"		Notes	

CHAMBERLAIN
U N I V E R S I T Y

Approvals

	APPROVED	APPROVED W/ CHANGES	DENIED	DATE	INITIALS
Stephanie Gallo	☐	☐	☐		
	☐	☐	☐		
	☐	☐	☐		
	☐	☐	☐		
	☐	☐	☐		

Pub Info

PRINT
Pub:
Issue:
Contact:

OOH
Title:
Location:
Prod Co:
Post Date:
Quantity:

3005 Highland Parkway | Downers Grove, IL 60515 | P: 630.512.8914 | F: 630.512.8888

FINAL CHECKLIST

	INITIALS	INITIALS
Chamberlain Address	☐	☐
Chamberlain Phone 888.556.8CCN (8226)	☐	☐
Chamberlain URL	☐	☐
3-Year BSN Copy	☐	☐
Full Accreditation	☐	☐
Institutional Accred.	☐	☐
Program Accred. BSN	☐	☐
Program Accred. MSN	☐	☐
Program Accred. DNP	☐	☐
State Approval (SCHEV)	☐	☐
TN State Disclosure (THEC)	☐	☐
IL Board of Higher Ed (IBHE)	☐	☐
Program Availability	☐	☐
Consumer Disclosure URL	☐	☐
Legal Line	☐	☐
Inventory Code	☐	☐
Production Code	☐	☐
Heat Map Check	☐	☐
Other:	☐	☐

Teaching Excellence Comprehensive Program

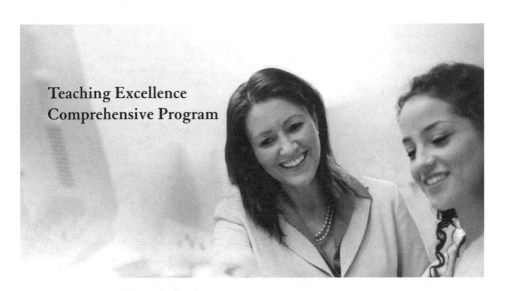

Teaching Excellence
Comprehensive Program

Dear Colleague,

Welcome to Chamberlain University.

The Teaching Excellence Comprehensive Program is a comprehensive, structured faculty development plan to successfully transition new faculty across their first year of teaching at Chamberlain. Included are the Teaching Excellence Foundations, an overview of skills and resources required for the academic role, and Teaching Excellence Curriculum, an index of required and recommended faculty development courses and resources. Timeframes for completion of required components are established to support you, our valued colleague, through a positive orientation experience. Joining a large institution such as Chamberlain can be a challenging experience, but it is also a highly rewarding one. During your first year of teaching, there will be skills to learn, colleagues to meet, and a new environment to explore. The Teaching Excellence Comprehensive Program was designed to make this process easier for you.

Please use this resource to establish regular and ongoing discussions with your campus leader, who will guide and support your successful transition to the College.

Thank you for your commitment to graduating extraordinary nurses! Again, welcome!

Laura Fillmore, DNP, MSN, RN, CNE
Director, Curriculum and Instruction
Center for Faculty Excellence
Chamberlain University – College of Nursing

Table of Contents

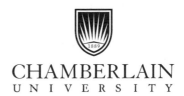

CHAMBERLAIN
U N I V E R S I T Y

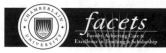

TEACHING EXCELLENCE COMPREHENSIVE PROGRAM

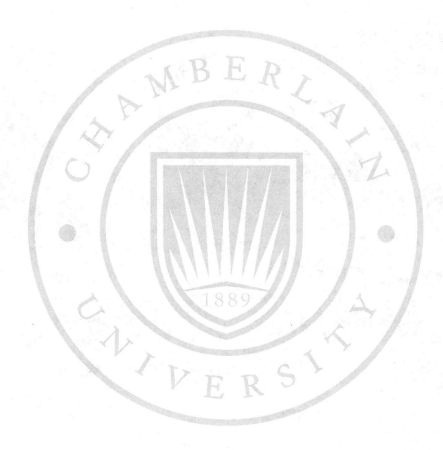

2

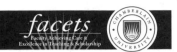

TEACHING EXCELLENCE COMPREHENSIVE PROGRAM

Teaching Excellence Foundations

Name:_____

Systems and Applications Training – 1st 30 days					
Activity	**Initial/Date**	**Activity**	**Initial/Date**	**Activity**	**Initial/Date**
Banner		Chatter		DocuSign	
DSAMS		Respondus		Voicemail	
Salesforce		Expensewire		Forwarding email to personal phone	
Shared Drive Access		Badge		Email signature	
SharePoint		Navigating Outlook and Lync		VPN	
DeVry Commons Navigation – 1st 30 days					
Bookmark: **thedevrycommons.com**		• IT Resources • Service Now		• Task Box (work flow) • AskHR • Thank a Colleague: Thanks a Million	
My Self Service • Benefits • Replicon • IPP • IDP • Personal profile • Talent profile		Career Development • Leadership center • Referral and bonus • Internal opportunities		Home Office Support • Ethics Compliance • Travel • Setting up SIREN	
Faculty Handbook – 1st 30 days					
Clinical Faculty Handbook – 1st 30 days					
Student Handbook – 1st 30 days					

3

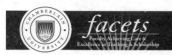

Teaching Preparedness – 1st 30 days					
Activity	**Initial/Date**	**Activity**	**Initial/Date**	**Activity**	**Initial/Date**
Academic Alignment		Learning Environment		NCLEX® Success	
Service to College (expectations) • Open Houses • Graduation		Faculty and student satisfaction surveys		Grading Essentials	
Faculty Dress Code		Office Etiquette		1:1 meetings with manager	

Faculty Observation – 1st 30 days					
Attend the following and observe effective use of *Master Instruction (MI)* concepts • Live lectures with at least two different faculty members • At minimum one live lab session • At minimum one open lab session • At minimum one live simulation and debriefing in the SIMCARE CENTER™ • At minimum one Center for Academic Success (CAS) workshop or tutoring session		Spend time with the course coordinator and faculty of assigned course to: • Prepare the course shell • Obtain course exams • Obtain course items (e.g. calendar) • Discuss assigned clinical rotation			

Faculty Support					
Course preparation completed (Refer to the Course Readiness Checklist job aid on the CFE portal)		Items to cover first day of class (Refer to the Course Readiness Checklist job aid on the CFE portal)		Resources for ongoing faculty support • Campus leadership • Center for Faculty Excellence • Business Process Analyst Team (for systems and applications types of issues) • Course Information Specialists (CIS) • Course Collaborative shells *Master Instruction (MI)* champions on campus	

Miscellaneous					

4

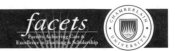

TEACHING EXCELLENCE COMPREHENSIVE PROGRAM

Teaching Excellence Curriculum

Required Center for Faculty Excellence Courses		
Completion Time Frame	**Required Course**	**Initial/Date**
Complete in first 14 days	CCN-101: Essential Guide for New Faculty Success (2 Hours) Username: CCN101-Success Password: CCN101-Success	Verified and reviewed: Date:_____ Initials:_____
Complete in first 120 days	CCN-130: Essential Guide for Advancing Faculty Success (6 Hours) Username: CCN130-AFS Password: CCN130-AFS	Verified and reviewed: Date:_____ Initials:_____
Complete in first 120 days	CCN-102: Essential Guide for Clinical Faculty Success (5 Hours) Username: CCN102-Clinical Password: CCN102-Clinical	Verified and reviewed: Date:_____ Initials:_____
Complete in first 180 days	CCN-110: *Master Instruction: **Chamberlain Care*** in Action (3 Hours) Username: CCN110-MI Password: CCN110-MI	Verified and reviewed: Date:_____ Initials:_____
Complete in first 240 days	CCN-115: *Master Instruction:* Evidence-Based Teaching (2 Hours) Username: CCN115-Teaching Password: CCN115-Teaching	Verified and reviewed: Date:_____ Initials:_____
Complete in first 365 days	CCN-120: Essential Guide for Scholarship (2 Hours) Username: CCN120-Scholarship Password: CCN120-Scholarship	Verified and reviewed: Date:_____ Initials:_____

Recommended Faculty Development Resources		
Complete in first 120 days	Nurse Tim Inc., Resources	Succeeding as a Nurse
		Promoting Academic Integrity
		Preventing Incivility: Proactive Solutions for the Classroom and Beyond
		Retention and Success: Creating a Student-Centered Culture Parts 1 & 2
		Looking for Evidence-Based Nursing Education
		NCLEX® Across the Curriculum Parts 1 & 2
Complete in first 365 days	Nurse Tim Inc., Resources	Concept maps in Nursing Education
		Delegation and Prioritization: Classroom and Clinical
		Clinical Reasoning Case Studies Across the Curriculum for NCLEX® Success
		Item Analysis Made Easy
		QSEN in Your Curriculum: Assumptions, Active Learning and Assessments
	CFE Portal Resources	Using Grading Rubrics; *Master Instruction* Classroom Observation Tutorial for Faculty

Access CFE required courses online at **nursingonline.chamberlain.edu**. The username and password are case sensitive.

Access the recommended "Nurse Tim" courses at **http://www.nursetim.com**. Chamberlain University's College of Nursing subscription code changes yearly (January). Locate current code at the "Learning Center" on CFE portal.

5

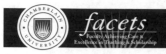

TEACHING EXCELLENCE COMPREHENSIVE PROGRAM

Teaching Excellence Concepts

FACETS Pathways e-Repository is a collection of valuable Reusable Learning Objects (RLOs) or digital resources to mediate faculty development. RLOs are thematically aligned to structure and sequence learning components, which address key topics for faculty teaching and development.

Faculty can use RLOs to personalize learning, taking into account experience, knowledge and learning goals. Faculty leaders can use RLOs to facilitate live or virtual, individual and/or collective discussions to advance teaching competencies. Complete all RLOs in one topic area for an in-depth exploration of essential content, or select individual RLOs to customize the learning experience based on learning style, special needs or level of competency. FACETS Pathways e-Repository facilitates the sharing and use of valuable RLOs to promote varied opportunities for enhanced learning experiences to meet individual, team and program needs.

Academic Alignment	Master Instruction	Grading Essentials	Academic Integrity	Student Performance Issues	Scholarship Essentials
CCN-101					
• Chamberlain's Curricula • Chamberlain's Evaluation Processes	Our Distinct Attributes: *Chamberlain Care®* and *Master Instruction* Pedagogy	Chamberlain's Evaluation Processes		• Our Chamberlain Community of Colleagues • Student Support Services	
CCN-102					
• Curricular Foundations • Student Orientation, Conferences & Patient Care Assignments	*Master Instruction (MI)*	• Clinical Evaluation Methods • Evaluation Strategies • Performance Assessment		• Legal & Ethical Issues • Performance Issues • Incivility • Student Misconduct • Academic Performance • Safe Performance • Just Report	
CCN-110					
	• *Chamberlain Care®* in Action Stories • Reflection Journal • *Master Instruction (MI)*: Teamwork & Reflection				
CCN-115					
Transformational Teaching	• Learning Theories • Transformational Teaching • Transformational Learning • Evidence-Based Teaching				
CCN-120					
					• Scholarship Essentials • Scholarship at Chamberlain
CCN-130					
• Purposeful, Pedagogical Teaching • Identifying Purposeful Learning Strategies • Wheel of Purposeful Learning					

TEACHING EXCELLENCE COMPREHENSIVE PROGRAM

facets
Faculty Achieving Care &
Excellence in Teaching & Scholarship

CHAMBERLAIN
UNIVERSITY

Notes

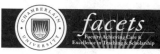

Master Instruction Classroom Observation Form

Master Instruction Classroom Observation is designed to advance the practice of *Master Instruction* through self-reflection and peer observation of campus-based and online faculty. Integral to *Master Instruction* is creating a positive, participatory learning environment through deliberate use of evidence-based strategies to foster deep student learning. Self and dialogic reflection expands perspectives to confront and resolve actual and desired teaching practices and facilitate successful student learning outcomes. The descriptors found in the left column are characteristics of *Master Instruction* and not specific tasks. Through self-reflection, the individual faculty member must interpret the criterion in the way that best meets the learning objective, content to be delivered and learning environment setting. Prior to the observation, the designated observer will review the self-reflection of the faculty member and then observe the faculty-student interaction and provide detailed feedback of the observation to promote professional development.

Directions

Faculty are required to validate completion of the *Master Instruction* Classroom Observation process twice per fiscal year. A Likert scale is used to record observation responses of each characteristic of *Master Instruction* to guide professional development only; it is not intended to serve as a performance evaluation. The observer must provide specific examples for each characteristic of *Master Instruction* to guide dialogue to advance the practice of *Master Instruction*. Following the observation, the observer will share their insights from the review with the faculty member in a private meeting. The purpose of this meeting is to expand perspectives through dialogic reflection to transform teaching practices. The faculty member will also reflect upon and rate his/her practice of *Master Instruction* to guide professional development.

Instructor	Instructor D#
Course	**Session**
Observer	**Observer Title**
Location	**Date of Observation**

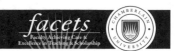

TEACHING EXCELLENCE COMPREHENSIVE PROGRAM

Content Management	
Relevant content, appropriately rigorous and applied to real-life concepts; explains how assignments and evaluation methods support course objectives; is prepared, current, credible, knowledgeable	Rate the extent to which this characteristic of *Master Instruction* is observed:

4. Exceeds Expected Results
- Outstanding performance almost without exception
- Consistently demonstrates exceptional results and behaviors above what is expected of the position

3. Fully Effective/Achieves Expected Results
- Solid performance
- Fulfills all expected results and behaviors
- Generates results above those expected of the position in some areas

2. Still Developing in Achieving Results
- Achieves results in some areas and requires development in other areas
- May need more consistency at times in achieving results
- Some additional development and improvement in results and/or behaviors is necessary in targeted areas

1. Does Not Fully Meet Expected Results
- Results in important areas are not being met
- Significant development and improvement in results and/or behaviors is necessary

Comments: (Include specific details)

Active Learning	Rating Scales
Engages students and holds their attention; challenges them to rethink their assumptions; uses multiple methods to promote learning	Rate the extent to which this characteristic of *Master Instruction* is observed:

4. Exceeds Expected Results
- Outstanding performance almost without exception
- Consistently demonstrates exceptional results and behaviors above what is expected of the position

3. Fully Effective/Achieves Expected Results
- Solid performance
- Fulfills all expected results and behaviors
- Generates results above those expected of the position in some areas

2. Still Developing in Achieving Results
- Achieves results in some areas and requires development in other areas
- May need more consistency at times in achieving results
- Some additional development and improvement in results and/or behaviors is necessary in targeted areas

1. Does Not Fully Meet Expected Results
- Results in important areas are not being met
- Significant development and improvement in results and/or behaviors is necessary

Comments: (Include specific details)

9

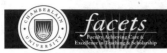

Relevance	Rating Scales
Application of materials; moves deliberately through Bloom's taxonomy; guides the use of scholarly work from the profession; uses evaluation methods that promote lifelong learning	Rate the extent to which this characteristic of *Master Instruction* is observed: 4. **Exceeds Expected Results** • Outstanding performance almost without exception • Consistently demonstrates exceptional results and behaviors above what is expected of the position 3. **Fully Effective/Achieves Expected Results** • Solid performance • Fulfills all expected results and behaviors • Generates results above those expected of the position in some areas 2. **Still Developing in Achieving Results** • Achieves results in some areas and requires development in other areas • May need more consistency at times in achieving results • Some additional development and improvement in results and/or behaviors is necessary in targeted areas 1. **Does Not Fully Meet Expected Results** • Results in important areas are not being met • Significant development and improvement in results and/or behaviors is necessary

Comments: (Include specific details)

Facilitation	Rating Scales
Uses a respond-extend-probe discussion model; allows students opportunities for trial/error feedback in advance of summative judgment of their work	Rate the extent to which this characteristic of *Master Instruction* is observed: 4. **Exceeds Expected Results** • Outstanding performance almost without exception • Consistently demonstrates exceptional results and behaviors above what is expected of the position 3. **Fully Effective/Achieves Expected Results** • Solid performance • Fulfills all expected results and behaviors • Generates results above those expected of the position in some areas 2. **Still Developing in Achieving Results** • Achieves results in some areas and requires development in other areas • May need more consistency at times in achieving results • Some additional development and improvement in results and/or behaviors is necessary in targeted areas 1. **Does Not Fully Meet Expected Results** • Results in important areas are not being met • Significant development and improvement in results and/or behaviors is necessary

Comments: (Include specific details)

TEACHING EXCELLENCE COMPREHENSIVE PROGRAM

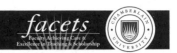

Integration	Rating Scales
Promotes learning outside the classroom; promotes curiosity with challenging questions, frequent feedback	Rate the extent to which this characteristic of *Master Instruction* is observed: 4. **Exceeds Expected Results** • Outstanding performance almost without exception • Consistently demonstrates exceptional results and behaviors above what is expected of the position 3. **Fully Effective/Achieves Expected Results** • Solid performance • Fulfills all expected results and behaviors • Generates results above those expected of the position in some areas 2. **Still Developing in Achieving Results** • Achieves results in some areas and requires development in other areas • May need more consistency at times in achieving results • Some additional development and improvement in results and/or behaviors is necessary in targeted areas 1. **Does Not Fully Meet Expected Results** • Results in important areas are not being met • Significant development and improvement in results and/or behaviors is necessary
Comments: (Include specific details)	

Classroom Environment	Rating Scales
Reinforces the learning agreement; fosters a learning spirit; promotes civility and professionalism	Rate the extent to which this characteristic of *Master Instruction* is observed: 4. **Exceeds Expected Results** • Outstanding performance almost without exception • Consistently demonstrates exceptional results and behaviors above what is expected of the position 3. **Fully Effective/Achieves Expected Results** • Solid performance • Fulfills all expected results and behaviors • Generates results above those expected of the position in some areas 2. **Still Developing in Achieving Results** • Achieves results in some areas and requires development in other areas • May need more consistency at times in achieving results • Some additional development and improvement in results and/or behaviors is necessary in targeted areas 1. **Does Not Fully Meet Expected Results** • Results in important areas are not being met • Significant development and improvement in results and/or behaviors is necessary
Comments: (Include specific details)	

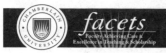

What was done especially well during the observation?

What are opportunities to transform teaching practices?

Self-reflection of the faculty member. Reflect upon and rate your practice of *Master Instruction*:

4. **Exceeds Expected Results**
   - Outstanding performance almost without exception
   - Consistently demonstrates exceptional results and behaviors above what is expected of the position

3. **Fully Effective/Achieves Expected Results**
   - Solid performance
   - Fulfills all expected results and behaviors
   - Generates results above those expected of the position in some areas

2. **Still Developing in Achieving Results**
   - Achieves results in some areas and requires development in other areas
   - May need more consistency at times in achieving results
   - Some additional development and improvement in results and/or behaviors is necessary in targeted areas

1. **Does Not Fully Meet Expected Results**
   - Results in important areas are not being met
   - Significant development and improvement in results and/or behaviors is necessary

12

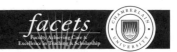

TEACHING EXCELLENCE COMPREHENSIVE PROGRAM

Clinical Faculty *Master Instruction* Observation Form

Master Instruction Clinical Observation is designed to advance the practice of *Master Instruction* through self-reflection and peer observation. Integral to *Master Instruction* is creating a positive, participatory learning environment through deliberate use of evidence-based strategies to foster deep student learning. Self and dialogic reflection expands perspectives to confront and resolve actual and desired teaching practices and facilitate successful student learning outcomes. The descriptors found in the left column are characteristics of *Master Instruction* and not specific tasks. Through self-reflection, the individual faculty member must interpret the criterion in the way that best meets the clinical learning objective, content to be delivered, and learning environment setting. Prior to the observation, the designated observer will review the self-reflection of the clinical faculty member and then observe the faculty-student interaction and provide detailed feedback of the observation to promote professional development.

Directions

Clinical faculty are required to validate completion of the *Master Instruction* Clinical Observation process twice per fiscal year. A Likert scale is used to record observation responses of each characteristic of *Master Instruction* to guide professional development only; it is not intended to serve as a performance evaluation. The observer must provide specific examples for each characteristic of *Master Instruction* to guide dialogue to advance the practice of *Master Instruction*. Following the observation, the observer will share their insights from the review with the clinical faculty member in a private meeting. The purpose of this meeting is to expand perspectives through dialogic reflection to transform teaching practices. The faculty member will also reflect upon and rate his/her practice of *Master Instruction* to guide professional development.

Instructor	Instructor D#
Course	**Session**
Observer	**Observer Title**
Location	**Date of Observation**

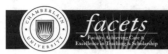

Content Management: Clinical Application of Course Concepts

• *Demonstrates preparedness*
• *Assists students to integrate course concepts with practical application*
• *Explains how clinical assignments and evaluation methods support course outcomes*

Rate the extent to which this characteristic of *Master Instruction* is observed:

4. **Exceeds Expected Results**
   • Outstanding performance almost without exception
   • Consistently demonstrates exceptional results and behaviors above what is expected of the position

3. **Fully Effective/Achieves Expected Results**
   • Solid performance
   • Fulfills all expected results and behaviors
   • Generates results above those expected of the position in some areas

2. **Still Developing in Achieving Results**
   • Achieves results in some areas and requires development in other areas
   • May need more consistency at times in achieving results
   • Some additional development and improvement in results and/or behaviors is necessary in targeted areas

1. **Does Not Fully Meet Expected Results**
   • Results in important areas are not being met
   • Significant development and improvement in results and/or behaviors is necessary

Comments: (Include specific details)

Active Learning

Rating Scales

• *Engages students and brings a spirit of creativity to clinical teaching*
• *Challenges student to rethink assumptions*
• *Uses multiple strategies to facilitate learning*
• *Facilitates clinical reasoning, critical thinking and problem solving*

Rate the extent to which this characteristic of *Master Instruction* is observed:

4. **Exceeds Expected Results**
   • Outstanding performance almost without exception
   • Consistently demonstrates exceptional results and behaviors above what is expected of the position

3. **Fully Effective/Achieves Expected Results**
   • Solid performance
   • Fulfills all expected results and behaviors
   • Generates results above those expected of the position in some areas

2. **Still Developing in Achieving Results**
   • Achieves results in some areas and requires development in other areas
   • May need more consistency at times in achieving results
   • Some additional development and improvement in results and/or behaviors is necessary in targeted areas

1. **Does Not Fully Meet Expected Results**
   • Results in important areas are not being met
   • Significant development and improvement in results and/or behaviors is necessary

Comments: (Include specific details)

14

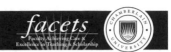

Relevance	Rating Scales

• Selects assignments based on student learning needs and course outcomes	Rate the extent to which this characteristic of *Master Instruction* is observed:
	
	4. **Exceeds Expected Results**
	  • Outstanding performance almost without exception
	  • Consistently demonstrates exceptional results and behaviors above what is expected of the position
	
	3. **Fully Effective/Achieves Expected Results**
	  • Solid performance
	  • Fulfills all expected results and behaviors
	  • Generates results above those expected of the position in some areas
	
	2. **Still Developing in Achieving Results**
	  • Achieves results in some areas and requires development in other areas
	  • May need more consistency at times in achieving results
	  • Some additional development and improvement in results and/or behaviors is necessary in targeted areas
	
	1. **Does Not Fully Meet Expected Results**
	  • Results in important areas are not being met
	  • Significant development and improvement in results and/or behaviors is necessary

Comments: (Include specific details)

Facilitation	Rating Scales

• Conducts preclinical conference to assess student preparedness and set priorities of care
 	
• Conducts postclinical conference to debrief student experiences
 	
• Promotes appropriate level of student autonomy for safe practice
 	
• Uses reflective learning
 	
• Provides effective formative and summative feedback to guide student clinical development
	Rate the extent to which this characteristic of *Master Instruction* is observed:
	
	4. **Exceeds Expected Results**
	  • Outstanding performance almost without exception
	  • Consistently demonstrates exceptional results and behaviors above what is expected of the position
	
	3. **Fully Effective/Achieves Expected Results**
	  • Solid performance
	  • Fulfills all expected results and behaviors
	  • Generates results above those expected of the position in some areas
	
	2. **Still Developing in Achieving Results**
	  • Achieves results in some areas and requires development in other areas
	  • May need more consistency at times in achieving results
	  • Some additional development and improvement in results and/or behaviors is necessary in targeted areas
	
	1. **Does Not Fully Meet Expected Results**
	  • Results in important areas are not being met
	  • Significant development and improvement in results and/or behaviors is necessary

Comments: (Include specific details)

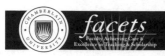

Integration	Rating Scales
• *Assists students to integrate classroom knowledge with practical application* • *Encourages reflection of learning to be applied in future*	Rate the extent to which this characteristic of *Master Instruction* is observed: 4. **Exceeds Expected Results** • Outstanding performance almost without exception • Consistently demonstrates exceptional results and behaviors above what is expected of the position 3. **Fully Effective/Achieves Expected Results** • Solid performance • Fulfills all expected results and behaviors • Generates results above those expected of the position in some areas 2. **Still Developing in Achieving Results** • Achieves results in some areas and requires development in other areas • May need more consistency at times in achieving results • Some additional development and improvement in results and/or behaviors is necessary in targeted areas 1. **Does Not Fully Meet Expected Results** • Results in important areas are not being met • Significant development and improvement in results and/or behaviors is necessary
Comments: (Include specific details)	

Clinical Learning Environment	Rating Scales
• *Reinforces the Student Pledge of Clinical Conduct* • *Promotes civility* • *Demonstrates professional behaviors consistent with moral, ethical, legal and regulatory principles and guidelines* • *Models and promotes nursing leadership through interprofessional collaboration* • *Establishes collegial relationship with agency/staff*	Rate the extent to which this characteristic of *Master Instruction* is observed: 4. **Exceeds Expected Results** • Outstanding performance almost without exception • Consistently demonstrates exceptional results and behaviors above what is expected of the position 3. **Fully Effective/Achieves Expected Results** • Solid performance • Fulfills all expected results and behaviors • Generates results above those expected of the position in some areas 2. **Still Developing in Achieving Results** • Achieves results in some areas and requires development in other areas • May need more consistency at times in achieving results • Some additional development and improvement in results and/or behaviors is necessary in targeted areas 1. **Does Not Fully Meet Expected Results** • Results in important areas are not being met • Significant development and improvement in results and/or behaviors is necessary
Comments: (Include specific details)	

16

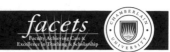

TEACHING EXCELLENCE COMPREHENSIVE PROGRAM

What was done especially well during the observation?

What are opportunities to transform teaching practices?

Self-reflection of the faculty member. Reflect upon and rate your practice of *Master Instruction:*

Rate the extent to which this characteristic of *Master Instruction* is observed:

4. **Exceeds Expected Results**
   - Outstanding performance almost without exception
   - Consistently demonstrates exceptional results and behaviors above what is expected of the position

3. **Fully Effective/Achieves Expected Results**
   - Solid performance
   - Fulfills all expected results and behaviors
   - Generates results above those expected of the position in some areas

2. **Still Developing in Achieving Results**
   - Achieves results in some areas and requires development in other areas
   - May need more consistency at times in achieving results
   - Some additional development and improvement in results and/or behaviors is necessary in targeted areas

1. **Does Not Fully Meet Expected Results**
   - Results in important areas are not being met
   - Significant development and improvement in results and/or behaviors is necessary

facets

Faculty Achieving Care &
Excellence in Teaching & Scholarship

TEACHING EXCELLENCE COMPREHENSIVE PROGRAM

Notes

TEACHING EXCELLENCE COMPREHENSIVE PROGRAM

facets
Faculty Achieving Care &
Excellence in Teaching & Scholarship

CHAMBERLAIN
UNIVERSITY

Notes

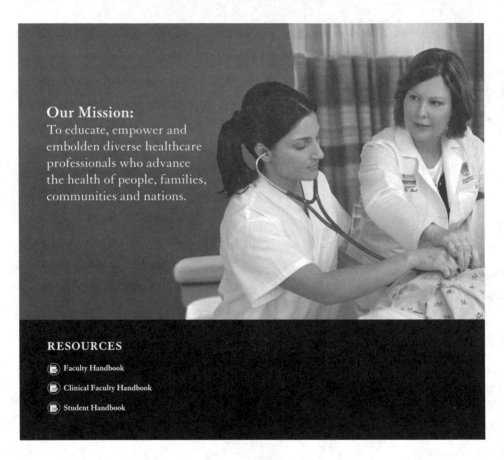

Our Mission:
To educate, empower and embolden diverse healthcare professionals who advance the health of people, families, communities and nations.

RESOURCES

- Faculty Handbook
- Clinical Faculty Handbook
- Student Handbook

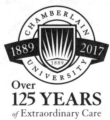

Over
125 YEARS
of Extraordinary Care

P-18413 A
Master Instruction Manual_Faculty Excellence_BW

| Date 07/19/17 | Printed At 100% | Agency PF |
| Time 5:00 PM | Round 6 | |

Job info

Element	Handbook	Pages	20 pg
Live	8.5" x 11"	Folded Size	
Trim	8.5" x 11"	VDP	☐
Bleed	.125"	Notes	

CHAMBERLAIN
U N I V E R S I T Y

Approvals

	APPROVED	APPROVED W/CHANGES	DENIED	DATE	INITIALS
Stephanie Gallo	☐	☐	☐		
	☐	☐	☐		
	☐	☐	☐		
	☐	☐	☐		

Pub Info

PRINT
Pub:
Issue:
Contact:

OOH
Title:
Location:
Prod Co:
Post Date:
Quantity:

FINAL CHECKLIST

	INITIALS	INITIALS
Chamberlain Address	☐	☐
Chamberlain Phone 888.556.8CCN (8226)	☐	☐
Chamberlain URL	☐	☐
3-Year BSN Copy	☐	☐
Full Accreditation	☐	☐
Institutional Accred.	☐	☐
Program Accred. BSN	☐	☐
Program Accred. MSN	☐	☐
Program Accred. DNP	☐	☐
State Approval (SCHEV)	☐	☐
TN State Disclosure (THEC)	☐	☐
IL Board of Higher Ed (IBHE)	☐	☐
Program Availability	☐	☐
Consumer Disclosure URL	☐	☐
Legal Line	☐	☐
Inventory Code	☐	☐
Production Code	☐	☐
Heat Map Check	☐	☐
Other:	☐	☐

3005 Highland Parkway I Downers Grove, IL 60515 I P: 630.512.8914 I F: 630.512.8888